Contents

Acknowledgments

It will be obvious to anyone who even dips into this book that it could not have been written without the substantial and penetrating contributions of the young people who use 42nd Street and of 42nd Street volunteers, workers, committee members and staff working for both funding and referring agencies. Particular acknowledgment is made to the support offered to this publication – and to the work of the agency – by Janet Batsleer, in her role as Chair of the Resource Management Committee. The supportive but tough way in which Alistair Cox, Sarah Dimmelow and Karina Nyananyo offered critical comment on endless drafts has also had a huge effect on the accuracy and quality of the content – though in the end, of course, I accept full responsibility for this and especially for the book's interpretations and judgments.

BERNARD DAVIES
October 2000

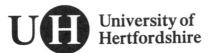 University of
Hertfordshire

College Lane, Hatfield, Herts. AL10 9AB

Learning and Information Services
College Lane Campus Learning Resources Centre, Hatfield

For renewal of Standard and One Week Loans,
please visit the web site **http://www.voyager.herts.ac.uk**

This item must be returned or the loan renewed by the due date.
The University reserves the right to recall items from loan at any time.
A fine will be charged for the late return of items.

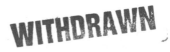

StreetCred?

Values and Dilemmas in Mental Health Work with Young People

BERNARD DAVIES

Published by

17–23 Albion Street, Leicester LE1 6GD.
Tel: 0116.285.3700. Fax: 0116.285.3777
E-mail: nya@nya.org.uk
Internet: http://www.nya.org.uk

In association with 42nd Street

ISBN 0 86155 237 7

© October 2000

Editor: DENISE DUNCAN
Cover photograph: LAWRIE PERRINS

YOUTH . WORK . PRESS
is a publishing imprint of the National Youth Agency

42nd. STREET

Founded in 1980, 42nd Street is a community-based mental health resource for young people under stress. Based in the city centre of Manchester, it offers a range of counselling and group work for young people aged 14 to 25 living in Manchester, Salford and Trafford. Community mental health workers take the service out into local communities to ensure the service can be accessed by young people who are usually overlooked by statutory mental health services.

Presenting problems include: isolation; depression; family conflicts; suicidal thoughts and attempts; repeated self-harm; sexual, emotional and physical abuse; concerns about medication; and problems caused by hospitalisation following a first breakdown.

42nd Street receives funding from Social Services Departments and Health Authorities in Manchester, Salford and Trafford; the Health Action Zone; the National Lottery; Comic Relief; and the Diana Fund. This funding is gratefully acknowledged.

The production of StreetCred? was made possible through a SmithKline Beecham Impact Award.

About the author

Bernard Davies first got involved in youth work in 1948 aged 13, as a member of a youth club and a Jewish Lads' Brigade unit. He went on to professional training via senior member and part-time leader and, after graduating with a history degree, took the one-year course for 'youth leaders and organisers' at University College Swansea during the year of Albemarle, 1958–59.

During the early 1960s he was a tutor at the National College for the Training of Youth Leaders and, after 18 months in the USA, for seven years ran a teacher-youth worker course at a mature student teacher training college in Lancashire. He served on advisory and review groups for the National Youth Bureau and Council for the Education and Training of Youth and Community Workers during the 1970s and 1980s and also served on a local authority education subcommittee and on local youth service review panels. His extensive experience of the voluntary sector includes chairing and being a member of local management committees and involvement as a local community activist. In 1983–84 he was president of the Community and Youth Workers' Union.

Throughout his career Bernard Davies has written extensively on youth work, the youth service and youth affairs. He contributed regularly to *New Society* in the 1960s and 1970s, co-authored *The Social Education of the Adolescent* with Alan Gibson, published in 1967, and has written pamphlets and a book, *Threatening Youth* (1986), on youth policies. Since taking early retirement as youth officer (training) from Sheffield Youth Service in 1992 he has acted as consultant for a number of voluntary organisations and local authorities including, with Mary Marken, carrying out a review of Sunderland Council's youth services.

Last year he wrote the two-volume *History of the Youth Service in England*, published by the National Youth Agency.

Preface

We hope that the themes that Bernard Davies has highlighted in this study of 42nd Street will reverberate in the thinking and planning of those who read it. We are proud of the fact that 42nd Street has survived the vicissitudes and crises of two decades. We are only too conscious of the sometimes conflicting demands involved in managing a determinedly value-based organisation – values which are about young people, mental health and the provision of an accessible community-based service.

When thinking about how to celebrate its 20th anniversary 42nd Street was always clear that it did not want a self-congratulatory historical account of the growth of an agency. We doubted the usefulness of this to a wider audience. What we asked for was an explicitly critical account of some key themes in the development of the service which might illuminate some of the dilemmas we face on a day-to-day basis. We hoped that this would also provoke a wider debate about how values may be sustained within services for young people at a time when pressures are more often about issues of contract compliance and conformity to externally determined funding objectives.

We would want to stress the importance of these themes at this time. Young people's voices need to be heard at a time when stress and related mental health issues are so central to their life experiences. We are conscious of the increasing numbers of young people who approach 42nd Street for help and of the parallel pressures experienced by many professional colleagues – in health, education, youth and social services and perhaps most acutely in residential provision. We don't think that 42nd Street necessarily provides a simple off-the-peg model for future provision. But we would argue that planners, managers and practitioners need to pay attention to the dilemmas and conflicts that Bernard Davies captures in this text if they are to create and support services for young people which are accessible and responsive to their needs.

Liz Green and Alistair Cox, 42nd Street Coordinators
October 2000

Introduction: Values into action

Driven by values

On first contact, what strikes an outsider about 42nd Street is, not surprisingly perhaps, what it is **doing** – particularly its wide range and unorthodox combination of methods and programmes. However, in describing itself as '*a community-based resource for young people under stress*', the agency itself lays at least as much emphasis on what it **believes** – both about what is possible and good for young people with mental health problems and about the best ways of tackling these.

This is not to say that since it was set up two decades ago it has not paid a great deal of attention to the pragmatics and the technicalities of its participation in the wider mental health world. Indeed, many of its internal debates still focus precisely on this interface and particularly on how to engage with it in young people's best interests. However, it has some bottom lines on how to define these which are sharply drawn, actively promoted – and fiercely defended. From these debates and exchanges, 42nd Street emerges as an organisation which, especially in today's welfare state climate, is to an unusual degree **value-driven**.

It is for this reason that this book focuses on 42nd Street's values – on the purposes and principles underpinning its work and its reasons for choosing these. It is therefore not mainly concerned with what 42nd Street actually does and how effectively and efficiently it does this when measured against those purposes and principles. Though the line is often not easy to draw, its primary aim is to unpack what 42nd Street means and understands by the key commitments embedded in these value positions.

Living history?

Indeed, the project out of which this book has arisen was deliberately given the working title 'Living History' in order to distance it from more mechanistic and ostensibly value-free models of historical and organisational analysis. It therefore attempts to do more than give an account of key events and shaping ideas, albeit located in the formal structures of the organisation and in the conditions in which it has operated over the past 20 years. Rather, to give this history a chance to **live**, it seeks to illuminate these inheritances from the past by exploring the value dynamics of the organisation **now** and how they express themselves within its **current** philosophy and culture.

The starting point therefore is not that as an agency 42nd Street 'just growed'. Instead, this study's working hypothesis has been that, in significant ways, it has been constructed out of an interplay of the values, intentions and actions of the **people** who have been involved in its work. This is most obviously reflected in the main source material for the book which – supplemented by observation of members', committee and team meetings and analysis of key documents and reports – appears as quotations from individual and group interviews carried out in the first half of 1999.

Well over fifty people contributed through these conversations, including young people, volunteers, paid workers (past and present, full and part-time, managerial, practitioner and administrative), committee members and representatives of funding and referral agencies. Within a loose structure of key prompt questions, all were encouraged to reflect on what they and 42nd Street as an institution mean – in theory and in practice – by such core concepts as 'young people', 'mental health', 'equal opportunities' and 'participation'.

Yet, to the extent that this book is a history, it does not assume that all is or has been for the best in the best of all possible worlds, with events always contributing naturally and inevitably to something called progress. Rather, a key test of its accuracy and authenticity will be how far, penetrating beyond the rhetoric, it provides descriptions and analyses which convey something of the untidiness, uncertainty, incompleteness and unresolved paradoxes intrinsic to complex helping processes.

Wider insights and messages

By explaining and re-presenting 42nd Street's value positions in this 'unfinished'[1] way, it is hoped that practitioners, managers and policy-makers in other health, social services, educational and welfare organisations will see reflected, and maybe even focus a little more sharply, something of themselves and their own practice and agencies. Ultimately, in fact, this aspiration has acted for me as the strongest stimulus for writing the book. This has, of course, needed to satisfy 42nd Street's expectation that – as it approaches its 20th anniversary – the book will provide a clear and accurate account of what it has sought and still seeks to stand for, and why. It has also needed to meet 42nd Street's wish that it will contribute something to the agency's credibility with an often sceptical and sometimes unsympathetic external environment.

However, my own most compelling motivation has been to explore the beliefs and intentions of an organisation which, after many years of involvement with young people, youth work and youth organisations, I have come to regard as distinctive. Hopefully, some investigation of that distinctiveness, though certainly **not** intended to produce simplistic models to imitate, might illuminate the complications of a vital field of practice – mental health provision for young people – and thereby prompt other providers into some critical (self-)reflection. More generally, I hope it will also clarify how value dilemmas, far from being the result merely of the failings of the individual managers or practitioners or of an organisation's technical arrangements, are inherent characteristics of policy and practice in any 'helping' agency.

Observing from within – and without

My emphasis on 42nd Street's distinctiveness perhaps betrays one other important starting point for this study: that I have not come to it as an entirely untainted observer. Insofar as objectivity is ever attainable in a human exercise

[1] See Thomas Mathiesen, *The Politics of Abolition*, Martin Robertson, 1974.

like this, the edge of my own has been somewhat blunted by my role over a number of years as an occasional external consultant with 42nd Street. Indeed, it was precisely because I had made the judgment that something unusual was going on here (or is it there?), especially in how value positions were articulated and their tensions confronted, that I agreed to take on the study in the first place.

Nonetheless, I have striven to remain a critical commentator on the organisation and especially to probe as open-mindedly as possible into, not just the statements 42nd Street makes on its values, but the contradictory ebbs and flows of expectation and interpretation which it has then to negotiate. Indeed, despite on occasions some inevitable nervousness and touchiness, guides and mentors from within 42nd Street have throughout urged me to allow my own outsider perspectives and voice to come through clearly and strongly, as an extra safeguard for the credibility of the analysis.

Structure

The book is thus constructed around what have emerged from the consultations as six core elements of 42nd Street's value position.

◆ **Chapter 1** (Young people and mental health) explores 42nd Street's choice to focus on 15 (now 14) to 25-year-olds. It examines how the agency sees young people's emotional, social and material condition, how it balances notions of adolescence-as-transition and adolescence-as-a-state-of-being in its own right, and the dilemmas of seeking to be 'young person centred'.

◆ **Chapter 2** (Mental health) considers the unease within 42nd Street with the notion of 'mental illness', tracing this back to the anti-psychiatry movement of the 1960s and 1970s. It explores its preference for working proactively with the notion that 'everyone has mental health' and its search for an alternative, based on social perspectives and collective responses, to the dominant medical model.

◆ **Chapter 3** (Professional approaches: youth work, therapy and informal support) discusses the rationale and the dilemmas of 42nd Street's multi-disciplinary methodology. Offering a continuum of opportunities embracing one-to-one counselling drawing on a range of psychotherapeutic perspectives, structured forms of therapeutic group work, informal youth work programmes and informal support for individuals, the chapter explores the resultant opportunities, tensions and choices for both users and staff.

◆ **Chapter 4** (Participation) looks critically at 42nd Street's commitment to user participation and empowerment – not just within its therapeutic relationships with young people but in the context of internal policy-making and in responding to local and national policy issues. Key focuses here are 42nd Street's efforts to establish a 'culture of empowerment' throughout the agency and, again, the often unavoidable dilemmas flowing from such a commitment.

◆ **Chapter 5** (Equal opportunities) discusses 42nd Street's understanding of equal opportunities and anti-discriminatory practice and its struggles here too with the accompanying dilemmas and contradictions. In particular, it explores what is involved in going beyond 'treating everyone the same' to a stance which positively embraces difference and diversity. It also examines 42nd Street's creation of black, women's, lesbian/gay and other named projects and posts to overcome the exclusion of oppressed groups while at the same time assuming an agency-wide responsibility for confronting the inequalities in young people's access and treatment.

◆ **Chapter 6** (Internal culture and external relations) focuses on 42nd Street as a voluntary sector organisation in a changed and changing welfare state environment. It looks at its commitment to internal policy-making, management and supervisory arrangements which, though specifically steering away from commitments to collectivity, are explicitly designed to be consultative and participative. It considers the implications of these arrangements for volunteers, part-time workers and members of the

Resource Management Committee (RMC) and the gains and potential risks of the organisation's increasing size.

◆ **Chapter 7** (Managing choices in a value-driven organisation) draws out lessons from the study for other health, social services, educational and welfare agencies.

Chapter 1: Young people and mental health

What stresses us out

Death/bereavement/losing someone close
Family/Home life **Divorce** Exams
Worrying about appearance
Household Chores **Money**
Peer Pressure Friends/arguing with friends
Losing things Boys/Men **Smoking**
Periods **Sex** Teachers *Racism*
Sexism Naughty little brothers/sisters
Coursework/deadlines Too Many Commitments
Competition **Revision** Time Pressures
Outside school activities **Illness** Orals/Speeches
Mondays Weight Problems
Prejudice **Insensitive people** **Bullying**
Future/preparing for life after school
Dilemmas Mums **Spots** Abortions
Rape *Cruelty to animals* **Crime**
Making hard decisions Pushy boyfriends
Tiredness **Pregnancy** **Clothes**
Dads*Models* Worried about old age *Abuse*
Sexuality Puberty **Alcohol** Pressure about sex
Sexually transmitted diseases Sexual violence Working
Drugs sexual abuse
Growing Up Employers Competitive friends
Driving lessons *The news* Violence **Police**
Diabetes Premenstrual Tension **Disabilities**
Stalking

Chapter 1: Young people and mental health

Why young people?

Schoolgirl Hazel W. had a preoccupation with death, the deputy Manchester City Coroner said today. Hazel, a 14-year-old pupil at ... County Secondary School had spoken many times about killing herself. Then, on June 9, Hazel threw herself off the top of a 14-storey block of flats.

Verdict: Suicide
[Manchester Evening News, June 1969]

This stark news report – almost, it seems, written yesterday – set the scene (and the tone) for *Young and Sick in Mind*, a 22-page pamphlet published in 1970 by the Manchester Youth Development Trust. Ten years later, having continued tragically to build up its evidence, the Trust spawned something like the 'walk-in consultation centre' which, *Young and Sick in Mind* concluded, was urgently needed in Manchester. It was this which became 42nd Street.

The new agency was thus assumed from the start to be a specialist service to young people experiencing stress – an **exclusive** focus which, as it has since emphasised, *'statutory health and social services find it difficult to provide'*. Indeed, within the maelstrom that is mental health provision in Britain, the usually rigid distinction made between childhood and adulthood rushes many young people into an adult status for which they are not ready – and which fails to recognise their particular, especially adolescent, needs. Too often they are then left to stumble unsupported through a bewildering no-person's land of services organised primarily around the presumption that if they are not a child they must of course be adult. Overnight, vulnerable and damaged minor in need of extensive state protection becomes mentally ill adult who must struggle to make sense of an often frightening adult psychiatric hospital.

By contrast, 42nd Street is uncompromising in seeing young people as young people and in holding onto this perspective as they move through the mental health challenges of their youth. As one funder put it: *'It offers a bridge between two sets of services, each of which often operates on, for young people, inappropriate assumptions.'* By striving to model good practice, 42nd Street also highlights the anomalies and limitations of much other mental health provision for this age group.

Such a tightly focused youth commitment is best explained as a response to an adolescent transition which, in this society, is rarely achieved without some level of stress. Adults largely – albeit increasingly mistakenly – still assume that, **because** they are adult, fixed compass points exist for plotting the direction of their lives. The lives of young people, by contrast, are marked – indeed, significantly defined – by high degrees of uncertainty and change which often extend to how they see and understand their very selves. Though often oversimplified, not always fitting easily together and too readily generalised to all in their teens, the causes of this flux nonetheless add up to a formidable set of 'developmental tasks'.

◆ Physical and hormonal changes of adolescence often produce some confusing emotional and psychological fall-out. This can be especially true for young people who are uncertain about their sexuality and/or who have experienced abusive or exploitative relationships which have left enduring personal scars.

◆ During these years, the young person has to find answers to a difficult yet urgent set of questions: 'Who am I?'; 'What is special, distinctive, about **me**?'; 'Where am I going in life?'. Past or current dysfunctions can again make the search painful and answers elusive.

◆ Many young people are increasingly having to make these adolescent transformations without any guarantee that even bottom-line requirements such as a decent income or independent accommodation will be met.

◆ Increasingly, too, the environment in which they have to make their choices is confusing, even alienating. In particular, while enticing with new and exciting opportunities, it often, at the same time, defines these – for example, using certain drugs, being sexually active – as illegal or, for young people specifically, morally wrong.

◆ These discriminatory social processes have different but often significant impacts on young women and young men, on young people depending on their class and on where they live, and on those who are black, gay, lesbian, bisexual and disabled.

◆ As a group as well as individually, young people have for long been metaphorically patted on the head and told: 'All will be well when you get to be an adult.' As well as disempowering and marginalising them, such patronising mind-sets also feed political, health and social welfare conventional wisdoms which label young people 'problematic'. The results increasingly are correction and punishment rather than interventions designed to discover and tap their strengths.

◆ The damaging effects of all this on young people's mental health are being documented. For example, as this book was being completed the influential Social Exclusion Unit produced statistics[2] which showed that:
  - in England and Wales 600 15 to 24-year-olds take their own life each year – that is, more than 10,000 since 1982;
  - up to 20,000 teenagers go to hospital each year as a consequence of deliberate self-harm; and
  - between the mid-1980s and the mid-1990s referrals for self-harm by young people increased by one-third.

◆ Where such stresses result in a diagnosis of 'mentally ill', young people are likely to meet some of the most stigmatising problem-definitions and punitive

[2] *National Strategy for Neighbourhood Renewal: Report of Policy Action Team 12: Young People*, Social Exclusion Unit, March 2000, 15,20.

responses, not least – as they themselves perceive it – by psychiatry and the mental health services generally.

While its precise form and degree of explicitness vary, a consensus around this kind of analysis of young people's condition and needs underpins – indeed drives – 42nd Street's commitment to providing a specialist mental health service for young people. One worker, for example, concluded that *'for young people adolescence is like a roundabout – going round and round with too many exits – what (are they) to do?'* while one of 42nd Street's funding agencies asserted bleakly that *'for young people the world today can be a bloody awful slippery slope'*.

'Young person centredness' and its dilemmas

Even while emphasising its steady focus on the special needs of young people, 42nd Street is nonetheless anxious to distance itself from assumptions that it is simply a service **for** young people whose style and content are determined only by those adults operating it. Indeed, by asserting that its goal is to be as 'young person centred' as possible, here as elsewhere it exposes its roots in that wider 1960s revolt against conventional psychiatry and the mental health establishment discussed more fully in Chapter 2.

However, at that time person-centred practice was gaining perhaps its most influential explicit expression in the work of Carl Rogers. His ideas penetrated deep into the thinking and above all the beliefs of successive generations of therapists, counsellors, educationists and other 'helping' professionals, asserting that a – perhaps the – key element of the helping process is *'an acceptance of this other person as a separate person with value in his own right; and ... a deep empathic understanding which enables me to see his private world through his eyes'*. [3]

Such a perspective now strikes, not only as unfashionable, but – for agencies reliant on state funding – as very risky. Current dominant (especially policy) imperatives are trained on moulding 'the youth of the nation' (a significantly

---

[3] Carl Rogers, *On Becoming a Person*, Constable, 1967, 34.

possessive phrase) into loyal and law abiding citizens, into dutiful husbands, wives and parents and into competent and flexible workers.

Nonetheless, the Rogerian preoccupations have been given explicit expression in 42nd Street literature and publicity at least since the mid-1980s. The 1996 annual report, for example, again emphasised '... *starting from respecting and valuing young people and acknowledging what they are experiencing in their lives'* – though by then it was firmly adding: *'This involves being sensitive to the wide variety of factors which may create pressures for young people from circumstances in their social context.'*

Practical and resource limitations can inevitably constrain such responsiveness – the waiting list for counselling, for example, was seen by one referral agency as a significant disincentive for some young people, one of whom has described it as *'sometimes a bit of a nightmare'*. Nonetheless, in providing their own appraisal of 42nd Street, users offered repeated, and grounded, endorsement of its young person centredness:

It hears your side of the story.
42nd Street ... is there for you when you need them.
Workers haven't just used me.
They don't judge you – but they don't write you off either.

For one volunteer '42nd Street was recommended ... because it took young people's needs as the starting point. They were the focus.'

As 42nd Street is well aware – and as, in a range of context, all subsequent chapters will illustrate – the **practice** of a notion like young person centredness is complex and often internally contradictory. Who, for example, has **the power** in young person centred relationships, especially when these are between professional and young person and professional and agency? (Rogers himself did not seem to acknowledge the presence of such dilemmas until quite late in his career.[4]) And, where conflicts emerge, how are balances struck between young

4 Carl Rogers, *On Personal Power*, Delta, 1977, pp3–4.

people's choices and workers' obligations to protect them from abuse or other harm or to challenge and even seek to change their perceptions and interpretations of what is happening to them?

Though not removing such dilemmas, when unpacked young person centredness in the 42nd Street context can be seen to be guided by some core, and tightly interrelated, values and principles. As recognised by young people, these at the very least include:

◆ Accepting the young person as they are:
'They make us feel welcome – want to know us ... They take you for who you are– they don't judge you.'

◆ Offering each young person respect:
'It hears your side of the story. I feel like a young person but I'm treated like an adult.'

◆ Starting where the young person is:
'They don't start by dishing out advice.'

◆ Searching out and building from the young person's strengths:
'42nd Street doesn't write you off. They don't put you down.'

◆ Working for and with the young person's autonomy:
'It's not like at school – it's not what they say you can do. You can do what you want ...'

◆ Legitimising the young person's feelings:
'I can bare my soul in the group if I want to ... can let out my anger.'

◆ Providing access by choice to a range of appropriate and flexible resources and facilities:
'The posters around tell you it's a youth area ... it's your area.'

Though they do not close the debates, such commitments do at least help to ground the notion of young person centredness in recognisable forms of practice.

How young is a young person – and how old?

It is not just commitments such as these, however, which expose 42nd Street to some of the unfinished dimensions of a specialist youth facility. Its very definition of young people brings its own dilemmas and choices.

For most of its existence 42nd Street has seen its youth target group as 15 to 25-year-olds. With the launch of its Children and Young People's Project, it extended this in 1996 in order to help fill *'gaps in the services for young people aged 14 to 16 years in Manchester'*. While successful in its outreach to this new group, within the broader spectrum of 42nd Street the project has been, in the words of the 1998 Annual Report, *'challenging ... and thought-provoking'*.

Such reactions are hardly surprising. Though all those falling within its declared age range might (just) identify themselves as young people, the fact that at 14 a user's needs are in significant ways different from those of a 25-year-old was always likely to stretch both 42nd Street's reach and its effectiveness. By dipping below the age of 16, it has had to amend its strict confidentiality policy, especially in the context of child protection. In some cases, too, and against long-standing 42nd Street assumptions, involvement with some users' families has become unavoidable while approaches to users' participation in the running of the organisation have also had to be reviewed (see Chapter 4).

Here as elsewhere some unintended as well as intended consequential costs (or at least tensions) have had to be balanced against the benefits of providing a service bridging the wider age range.

Adolescence as transition

For negotiating these dilemmas, 42nd Street's approach is underpinned by influential **unifying** conceptions of youth. Most explicitly, these emphasise transition as central to its definition and to young people's own subjective experience of this period of their lives. Within 42nd Street this is variously described by workers, volunteers and representatives of external agencies as *'a journey, a cross-over, a passage from dependent child to independent adult, moving through the universal experience of adolescence towards the positive goal of adulthood.'* It is a movement which, it is recognised, individuals will undertake at different speeds and some of whose defining features will be experiment and unpredictability.

Thus, one worker saw it as important to accept that *'young people are trying out many versions of themselves'* while another commented that, for young people *'as soon as they are through one door, everyone moves on'*. Moreover, positive outcomes from this transitional phase are certainly not assumed to be guaranteed. Perhaps significantly, it was left to two of 42nd Street's external funders to note that *'if things go wrong there can be damage later – the problems can be more fundamental'*; and that *'getting in early can stop serious trouble later'*.

The here-and-now of adolescence

This interpretation of adolescence-as-transition is not always helpful, however, least of all for developing sensitive and appropriate forms of service delivery. As one 42nd Street user noted: *'Other organisations put you down – give you crap because you're a young person. They just tell you it's a phase you're going through.'* One worker described attitudes 'out there' as perpetuating the assumption that *'young people's problems can't be that severe. After all, they'll grow out of them, won't they?'*

Yet, for the young person who is actually negotiating the adolescent years their experiences are not merely stations along a track heading inexorably towards the one desirable destination of being 'grown up'. These experiences often have validity – indeed value – in their own right, for what they mean **now**.

Here, some well-founded western perspectives on childhood can be illuminating.

Though now too politically inconvenient to shape educational and social work priorities in the way it did in the 1960s, substantial evidence still exists, for example, that for young children the play activities which are so prominent in their lives are much more than mere pastimes. Not only do these advance important social and practical learning. Through them, the child comes to know more clearly who she or he is in relation to others, and they allow vital forms of self-expression to occur and self-concepts to be strengthened. Such insights also help to explain why this stage in the life cycle is described as child**hood** – a statement of **being**, an implicit assertion of the importance of the here-and-now.

In contrast, adoles**cence**, in common with words such as 'confluence' and 'transience', emphasises movement and flow, thereby reinforcing the adult preoccupation with what the young person is to **become**. Though in this country with little distinguishable impact, it was precisely to help loose those working with young people from this kind of conceptual trap that Henry Maier, an American childcare specialist, suggested as long ago as 1965 that this stage in the life cycle be conceptualised as '**adolescenthood**'.[5]

Certainly for young people, and not least for young people experiencing serious levels of disappointment and stress, **now** can impact only too powerfully – and in its own right. A broken teenage relationship is much less significant for how it might affect the later choice of a life partner – even assuming that that is the young person's aspiration than for the disappointment and self-doubt it causes immediately. Daily humiliation at school matters today for how it affects the young person's standing among friends or next week's examination preparation – and not just for its potential damage to long-term career trajectories. The same is true of a failed job interview which may mean still not having work or enough money. As well as bestowing weighty baggage to carry into later life, the 'mental illness' label is also liable, in the present, to shape self-image and personal relationships in powerful ways.

---

[5] Henry Maier, 'Adolescenthood', *Social Casework* (US), Vol. 46, No. 1, 1965.

The priority of the present was vividly asserted by the young people whose testimony provided the core evidence of *Who's Hurting Who?*, 42nd Street's research report on suicide and self-harm. Within this, the future was rarely in sight and was certainly not dominant. Even the past got comparatively little direct attention. Instead, the young people stayed unrelentingly in the here-and-now, often confronting it with a searing honesty and intensity:

'When I cut myself, things which are overwhelming you in your daily life aren't, just for five minutes, maybe an hour, or however long I think about cutting myself and doing it and all that after care ... It used to give me a few hours break.'

'I'd been in a situation I wasn't happy with and I didn't know what to do and I was really miserable and fed up and wanted to be dead and I thought I'm not going to kill myself so what's the next best thing so I can just get out of this situation for a few hours.' [6]

Within 42nd Street, this concern with the now of adolescence is underpinned by other core principles and approaches, explored in detail in later chapters. As far as possible definitions of stress are applied which are everyday and non-diagnostic – as arising, for example, out of bullying or experiences of oppression. Stress triggers are recognised too which, though conventionally defined as adult, intrude very directly and damagingly into the lives of many young people: poverty and unemployment, bereavement, physical illness, being a parent, experiences of emotional stress and breakdown resulting in hospitalisation (see Chapter 2).

Without ignoring the impact of adolescent transition, considerable emphasis is therefore placed within 42nd Street practice on helping young people to secure a better future for themselves by encouraging and supporting them to do hard and often urgent emotional work, not just on the past, but also on the present (see Chapter 3). What is less clear, at least in comparison to the explicit commitments made to adolescence-as-transition, is how explicitly and confidently this focus is

[6] Helen Spandler, *Who's Hurting Who?: Young people, self-harm and suicide*, 42nd Street, 1996.

conceptualised and articulated as a valued dimension of the work.

Youth unbroken

In arguing for a specialist youth-focused service, 42nd Street emerged from two interlocking convictions – that:

◆ especially in the mental health field, a bureaucratically imposed split at 16 in the adolescent transition makes no sense at all; and

◆ given the scars so often left by deeply stressful experiences, young people may need that consistent support even to the age of 25.

Such commitments are not without their inherent tensions – indeed, these seem still to dissuade most mental health agencies from spreading themselves across such an age range. For 42nd Street, however, seeing a young person through to their own best stab at adulthood while, paradoxically, continuing to work with them as young people **now** has remained central to its philosophy and practice.

Chapter 2: Mental health

It was quiet,
The room was quiet, everything was.

She switched on her music,
the volume was all consuming.
The paper-thin-blade laughed,
As her arm, silent, lay down.

Then to its job.
Noise was released,
Great shouting and fighting
and choking and crying
and pleading and begging
and anger and hate
screamed down her arm.

They all laughed
As they dripped off her hand,
free to play and shout
and laugh and fight-
Bright colours, and warm.

The mouths on her arm
were still screaming
and crying and screaming.
She tried to shut them up
with a towel.
But they bit into her
and still they screamed
and would not let go of her,
their lips curled back to show
bared teeth, snarling.

By day she muffled their cries
with a sleeve,
'til their scared lips
sealed silent shut.

Chapter 2: Mental health

What terms shall we use?

Underpinning 42nd Street's 20-year history has been a determination to give young people maximum protection from the stigmatising cultural and organisational meanings attached to the notion of 'mental health': from *'the stereotype of "being mad", the negative images it produces, its bad press'*. One user's fear – that *'people outside see mental health as meaning loopy'* – was confirmed by a referring agency which highlighted *'how keen young people are to say: I'm not mental.'*

Indeed, the current of doubt about the very term mental health running through 42nd Street's thinking seems during the 1990s to have shifted its public self-presentation: from *'a community mental health resource (or service) for young people'* to *'a community based resource for young people under stress'*. Paid and unpaid workers still talk of *'a struggle to find a language, of hesitating to use the term'* – even of avoiding it.

The bequest of anti-psychiatry: grappling with the politics of mental health

At root, this semantic nuancing is not just prompted by a distaste for certain words and images. In collision are contending conceptions of mental health and especially the values underpinning them. Within this, occasionally expressed directly, usually merely lurking, is an analysis of mental health ideology and practice reaching back at least to the 1960s when critics like R. D. Laing, David Cooper and Erving Goffman injected ideas into the culture of mental health provision which continue to exert their influence.

Oversimply, these sought first to grasp, and then to work from, the mentally ill's own experience of mental illness. By highlighting the often debilitating effects of the disease labels attached to 'patients', these perspectives repeatedly redefined 'helpers' as at least part of the sick person's problem. They also questioned how far such labels were genuine scientific descriptions of ill-health rather than the subjective creations of powerful medical practitioners.

Some at the forefront of this attempted 'anti-psychiatry' counter-revolution also found 'truths' in the mentally ill person's experience as valid as those provided by the sane. In doing this they sometimes strayed so far from the scientific into the romantic and the mystic that they too lost credibility, even with some sympathisers. Nonetheless, in at least one key respect they left a lasting mark. They changed the **political** discourse within mental health: indeed, some would argue, they created such a discourse where none had existed before. Most specifically, they sought to shunt power in patients' direction, in the process sowing unfamiliar doubts about the infallibility of the doctor.

Inevitably, this assault on the bastions of medical-model psychiatry was largely repulsed. Nonetheless, it left fissures in the structure through which more critical organisations have been able to infiltrate sometimes dangerously subversive ideas and ways of working. Three-plus decades on, 42nd Street can in part be understood as one such Trojan horse.

Unlike many powerful institutions and professions, 42nd Street has consistently acknowledged the power at its disposal as an inescapable reality in its transactions with users. Indeed, as we shall see later, sustaining young people's responsibility for and power within their own lives remains one of its core values. However, accepting the difficult judgments and choices required, it has sought, too, to treat such power as a potential resource to be used **by workers** in young people's interests. As one worker put it, its commitment is *to holding authority helpfully: 'This is frequently displayed in our assumption of an advocacy role with a range of mental health agencies to address complaints or gain access to alternative treatments. Most starkly it is required at the rare moments when a decision has to be made to break confidentiality, because concerns about a young person's safety override their expressed wishes.'*

Mental health: Normal and universal

Though now something of an orthodoxy, another of the anti-psychiatry insertions from the 1960s has been the proposition, verbalised by one 42nd Street worker, that *'everyone has mental health'*; or, as one volunteer expressed it: *'No-one is too well to use the services of 42nd Street.'* Here, its starting point as a youth agency is that *'working with young people (inevitably) means working with their mental health needs'.* As one funder acknowledged, this assumes that *'often we're dealing with the very ordinary, with very ordinary young people'* who, as well as dealing with normal adolescent feelings and choices, can also, as we have seen, be overtaken by such familiar adult life crises as illness, bereavement and fracturing family relationships.

On the grounds that, in dealing with such traumas *'young people may not yet have reached the major mental health problems of the full-time psychiatric patient'* (funder), this perspective has clearly pointed 42nd Street towards preventive *'demand-led rather than crisis-led'* strategies (worker). This same emphasis seemed to be echoed in one referring agency's passing reference to 42nd Street's adoption of a *psycho-educational model*. Indeed, through some of the agency's ongoing programmes, workers and volunteers explicitly see themselves as working to help young people reach calmer, personally developmental waters by breaking cycles of stress→isolation→exclusion→stress→psychiatric illness.

Such perspectives were given their most systematic test by 42nd Street between 1993 to 1996, through its Education Project. With explicit preventive aims, this encouraged young people in schools, youth projects and at specially convened events to consider what (potentially or actually) endangered their emotional stability and confidence and how they might respond. Most of the project's programme focused on the everyday experiences of stress identified by young people themselves through anonymous questionnaires. Bullying and other tensions in peer relationships, conflicts with parents, examination pressures, racial and sexual harassment, coming out as lesbian or gay and other people's attitudes to their disability repeatedly emerged from these enquiries as young people's most emotionally wearing and threatening concerns.

Mental health needs were thus again substantially (though not exclusively) defined as what young people said they were – a position which still underpins agency-wide practice. Often, indeed, this gets articulated in young people's own vernacular – as catering for those who are **'stressed out'**, **'having a hard time'**, **'not having a lot going on for them'** or being **'pissed off'**.

Engaging with the medical model

Mental health services: some inescapable realities

Yet, despite its emphasis on the normality and universality of young people's mental health needs as seen from their perspective, responding to (often serious) breakdown and illness still makes up 42nd Street's core business. It thus finds itself inescapably drawn into a complex engagement with 'medical model' conceptions of and provision for mental health – into an implicit, if not explicit, 'world view' which is, at root, behaviourist. Here, professional methodologies are dominated by clinical diagnoses and treatment regimes involving the administration of drugs to cure or alleviate conditions of ill-health, with balances of power normally tipped strongly against 42nd Street's users.

Clearly, such perspectives and practices do not sit easily with the holistic, person-centred commitments constantly asserted within 42nd Street as at the heart of its approaches – a discomfort which is often openly acknowledged. As one worker put it: *'How okay is it to say: "The doctor's doing a good job" or "The drugs prescribed are really right"? ... There's a much looser consensus (within 42nd Street) around mental health than around young people.'*

Though more positive, another remained ambivalent: *'Some of us are more anti-psychiatry than others. I'm not for throwing the baby out with the bath water. There's a place for the medical model. Drugs can be useful.'*

One funder also seemed to recognise – even perhaps to some degree share – this ambivalence, concluding that *'though 42nd Street is often seen as having no time*

for medical models ... it would seek (medical treatment) for young people needing it.'
However, most external interests exert a strong and decisive pull on the
organisation towards medical perspectives on mental health. One referring
agency for example stressed that *'though we look at the whole person, their
housing, their income – ultimately we're looking for a diagnosis, for treatment'*. Even
more powerful, however, are the drag effects of money if only because, in the
mental health field, this is most often likely to follow what one funder called
'problems which are severe and enduring'.

Within 42nd Street, such notions – particularly that of severity of need – are
subject to sharp and ongoing debate. What is this? How do you recognise its
changes over time and what do you do about young people who move in and out
of such a state? What degree of severity should qualify a young person for access
to 42nd Street's services? Must this be deep-seated or does it also cover the
transitional stresses of adolescence? And again: whose answers should count
most – the professional's or the young person's?

The realities of user demand

What such exchanges do help to confirm is that agency responses to these pull
factors are strongly reinforced by push pressures exerted by young people
themselves. As one worker pointed out, these surface even from within a
commitment to accentuating the normal and the universal: *'In the midst of what
they may think of as a "brilliant" life, some young people who come here may just
not feel very confident – may somehow feel they could be doing better. It doesn't mean
their life is crap but it has to be taken seriously. It could hide something really serious
like abuse, or they might really be quite depressed.'*

For 42nd Street, such cautions are well taken. A majority of its membership bring
with them on-going experiences of serious trauma, often with medical labels
already firmly attached and their 'mental health' defined largely by its absence.
Users themselves are often only too clear about this, asserting (including at
public events) that though their encounters with hospital or GP may have been
bad, their complaints are more about insensitivity and lack of care than about

being treated medically. For 42nd Street, doctrinaire stances on the medical model are thus hardly an option, as one young person made clear: *'It felt important that a psychiatrist was prepared to listen to me.'*

Operating at the sharp end

Though it is self-consciously working across a complex spectrum of shades of personal distress, for much of its time 42nd Street is therefore operating close to its sharp end. In the words of one worker, much of its work is with *'young people with ... sad lives out of control ... (and) experiences of horrifying encounters with the services'*. More specifically, this means that *'42nd Street recognises that suicide and self-harm exist – unlike many other agencies like GPs'* (volunteer). External agencies explicitly state that they refer young people *'struggling with problems over sexuality, abuse, depression'*, not least because it employs professionally qualified counsellors. For one young person, the point about 42nd Street was that *'it has stopped me drinking'*.

The evidence gathered for *Who's Hurting Who?* constantly reinforced this picture, and not only in relation to the extent and severity of the self-harm which 42nd Street users were surviving:
'I was in a violent relationship and had been attacked by this guy who'd been an absolute bastard to me.'

'I was abused in a car and sometimes I get flashbacks; it's like I'm reliving it.'

'I got beaten up by mum's new husband and by his mum and dad.'

Young people as survivors

In dealing even with such deeply troubled young people, 42nd Street continues to emphasise normalisation. Not only does it strive **not** to relate to users as if they are **defined** by their mental health condition. It also in effect presses **them** not to own or act solely on such self-images and self-definitions. As different users put it: *'I've been stigmatised for having mental illness ... But not at 42nd Street.*

Only not at 42nd Street'; and: *'I've only once been persuaded at 42nd Street to go to hospital'.*

The emphasis is thus placed not on young people as victims but as survivors, and on their healthy characteristics and resources for dealing both with the here-and-now and with the transition into a satisfying adulthood. The agency sets out unashamedly to exploit *'young people's resourcefulness and dignity for their survival* (worker); *to enable them to use their own coping mechanisms, develop so they take responsibility for themselves* (volunteer)'.

In the wider mental health world in which 42nd Street moves such stances can leave the organisation misunderstood – and sometimes badly exposed. What are we doing, key power-brokers and purse-string holders might ask, supporting an agency which, though undoubtedly grappling with young people's serious and long-term mental health problems, at the same time prioritises early support to young people experiencing everyday adolescent stress? By questioning not just the terminology but more importantly the mind-sets shaping conventional medical-model mental health responses, 42nd Street is constantly in danger of offering up hostages to fortune which at any moment might be seized by interests increasingly focused on measurable medical 'outcomes'.

Towards a social model of mental health

Potentiality not deficiency

Perhaps unavoidably, some of 42nd Street's attempts to propound alternatives to the medical model and what it produces are expressed in negative terms: as *'a non-medical model; a non-medical approach; against labelling; non-pathologising; non-oppressive; against involuntary treatment; a non-hospital, non-institutional, non-diagnostic service'.*

Most positively and strategically, however, alternatives to the medical model are embodied in a conception of 'mental health' which substitutes a potentiality model of youth – what an admin worker explained as *'seeing young people in a holistic way'* – for the disease/deficiency perspectives which inform so much medical thinking. This model particularly focuses on each young person's capacity for personal and interpersonal growth via greater self-awareness and understanding (so that, according to one user, *'you feel worthy of yourself'*); and on improving their mental health through increased insight into and ability to deal with relationships with family members, partners, friends and other key actors in their lives.

From individual to structural explanations of problems

Despite their clear developmental emphases, by emphasising change in the individual young person's 'inappropriate' attitudes, behaviour and lifestyle, even these perspectives carry the risk of, at least implicitly, 'blaming the victim'. Such explanations of young people's problems sit awkwardly with 42nd Street's wider analyses of their current difficulties which are seen as having often deep structural roots, particularly in unsympathetic and even exploitative economic, social and political institutions largely beyond their individual influence.

Individually focused conceptions of mental health are therefore actively supplemented within 42nd Street by ones which recognise how far this (or its absence) is determined by the material conditions which, often brutally, shape and constrain personal choice and response, not least for young people. Starting from such a definition, achieving adequate income, decent accommodation and social and leisure opportunities and full legal and civil rights are all seen as vital to any young person's mental health or its restoration.

Towards collective responses

These (still largely individually focused) responses also act as building blocks for more collective interventions which are often (deliberately) interwoven closely into 42nd Street's commitment to young people's participation (see Chapter 4). Many of these are specifically aimed at influencing key mental health policies, locally and nationally. These have included:

◆ influential involvement in mental health service reviews in Manchester, Salford and Trafford;

◆ being consulted by the Audit Commission;

◆ contributing to the Mental Health Foundation National Inquiry into young people's mental health needs; and a Mind enquiry into mental health services; and

◆ running conferences on suicide and self-harm and on gay and lesbian issues which attracted national audiences.

The social action pilot projects being developed within 42nd Street also contribute to these struggles to construct a more socially oriented model of mental health. As spelt out by the Centre for Social Action at De Montfort University in Leicester, a social action approach places young people's individual and collective empowerment at the heart of everyday practice. In the case of 42nd Street, this includes its therapeutic group work practice as well as more obviously policy-oriented and political activities. It thus roots itself in three key principles:

◆ a recognition that **all** people have the capacity to create social change and that they should be given the opportunity;

◆ professionals work in partnership with people in the community; and

◆ the agenda is handed over to the people themselves. [7]

Taken together, 42nd Street has gone some way to clarifying what a social model of mental health might mean, and become, by committing itself both to confronting individual young people's material problems and building up their

[7] Jennie Fleming, Mark Harrison and David Ward, 'Social action can be an empowering process: a response to the scepticism of Monica Barry', *Youth and Policy*, 60, Summer 1998.

collective strength for changing their own immediate personal circumstances **and** mental health provision generally. However, given that what is being sought here is a framework of values, principles and methods capable of challenging the dominance of the medical model, is this **concept** adequate? Deliberately or not, might it not do more to mystify rather than clarify key underlying issues and choices? Since what is repeatedly being highlighted is a need to tip power balances towards users within the mental health world, perhaps what is actually being sought is, unmasked, an openly **political** model of mental health practice.

Beyond a medical model of mental health

42nd Street is of course very far from alone in its unease with medical model conceptions of mental health and in particular their deeply embedded individual pathology analyses and often overwhelmingly behaviourist presumptions and prescriptions. The challenge, however, is to move from such agonising to action and in particular – with like-minded partners – to developing a coherent **working** alternative capable of weakening the dominance of the medical model.

Since the murder of Jamie Bulger by two other very young children, the climate has changed, with – at least in this country – something called 'the evil personality' being reinstated as **the** populist and indeed often political explanation of why a tiny minority of young people act in tragic and apparently irrational ways. The auguries for building the kind of alternative project on which 42nd Street is embarked are therefore not good. Indeed, the resurgence of these demonising perspectives might even be taken as a warning of the possible loss as well as gain resulting from too comprehensive a dismissal of the medical model.

Nonetheless, 42nd Street can be seen as at least one agency which – actively and constructively – has gone in search of an alternative to the cruder versions of such a model – by, for example:

◆ asserting a core respect for young people's own perceptions and evaluations of their situation, needs and especially the service they are getting; pressing that these be taken seriously; and routinely using them to justify its own bids for funds;

◆ emphasising structural explanations of what, often routinely, young people are experiencing;

◆ assuming their potential for finding their own way, individually and collectively, to some legitimate responses; and

◆ seeking to integrate more systematic social action strategies and tactics into some of its group work programmes, including providing access to other, explicitly political and campaigning, organisations.

In the political arenas of mental health, it is in these grounded ways, it would seem, that some of the balances of power may begin to be tipped towards more holistic, humanistic and socially conscious models of mental health – and, thereby, in favour of young people themselves.

Chapter 3: Professional approaches – youth work, therapy and informal support

One-to-one support – My lifeline

My life two and a half years ago seems like a lifetime ago to me now. What I can remember is that I was an empty shell – all smiles on the outside but on the inside I was screaming and screaming LOUD. I just didn't want to live. The only release I had for all of these feelings was to self-harm. When it all got too much for me I would try to end my life by taking overdoses. But, I remember saying to myself, 'There must be more to life for me'.

I remember getting my first appointment at 42nd Street. I thought, 'right that's it – in two months my life will be sorted out'!

Chapter 3: Professional approaches – youth work, therapy and informal support

One-to-one support – My lifeline

My life two-and-a-half years ago seems like a lifetime ago to me now. What I can remember is that I was an empty shell – all smiles on the outside but on the inside I was screaming and screaming LOUD. I just didn't want to live. The only release I had for all of these feelings was to self-harm. When it all got too much for me I would try to end my life by taking overdoses. But, I remember saying to myself, 'There must be more to life for me'.

I remember getting my first appointment at 42nd Street. I thought, 'right that's it – in two months my life will be sorted out'! I must of thought the counsellor had a magic pill or something. I wish it was that easy. Anyway, I remember being so nervous, like waiting outside the head teacher's office at school. But I felt I could trust the counsellor I met right there and then, which was so important to me.

The issues for me were childhood abuse, physical violence, self harm and suicide attempts. I was a real mess. I had no confidence or self belief. I was worthless and that was it. But the counsellor helped me to explore this, and why I felt this way. When it was all broken down week by week, I began to see that this was what other people thought of me. I had never been allowed to actually think for myself. I didn't know what to do, as all my life had been for someone else. Not one part of my life had been for me, and 22 years is a long time to live only to please others.

It was hell finding out all of this. I remember wanting to have never found it out, to have never come to 42nd Street. What you don't know can't hurt you, right? No – wrong! I was hurting so bad on the inside that I had to release it, and the only way I could was to self-harm, that was my only way of coping with these DEMONS inside.

But where do I go from here? It was like someone had placed me in a jungle, without a map, compass, or anything to find my way or make deciding easy. I had to fend for myself and make my own decisions. It was so scary. How do I think for myself and what is it I want?

I became actively involved in 42ⁿᵈ Street. I spoke at conferences, wrote an article for a magazine, attended a child sexual abuse rally, helped to run a suicide and self-harm awareness day and co-facilitated a women-only suicide support group called Staying Alive.

Now I am going to be all on my own for the first time in my new life. This is scaring me a little really. But the counsellor tells me I'm a much stronger person now. I've overcome some of my most feared DEMONS inside of me, and come out on the brighter side ready to fight all over again. There is just no way to keep me down now – not for long anyway. I just won't let it. Look out world here I come!!

I've only mentioned a small amount of the one-to-one work I've done. My past is still a GREY area NOT BLACK BUT STILL A DARKER SHADE IN MY LIFE and my past still causes me great pain. I have to still work on this a lot. SO I don't want to give the impression that having counselling is an easy option. It's a big step and a gamble. As you change, you may lose people. You are not the same person they are comfortable with. So your whole world really gets turned upside down and back to front … It takes a lot of courage to do this and strength and determination. But once you find these qualities you will have them with you for life.

In search of multi-disciplinary practice

'It is 1981. A representative of one of 42ⁿᵈ Street's funders takes out a newspaper cutting from his file. Describing the tragic death of a young man, its implied "line" is that in some way his suicide was the fault of the local voluntary agency to which he had briefly turned for help. The report makes no mention of the psychiatrists or social workers who had been seeing the young man for some time. From the funding agency the message seems to be: "Isn't 42ⁿᵈ Street going to get itself into a similar mess?".'

Throughout the 1970s the Manchester Youth Development Trust's detached youth workers reported demands from young people for urgent help with their mental health difficulties. The Trust's efforts to set up an appropriate specialist service were blocked by powerful professional interests canvassing often contradictory arguments. Young people, Trust staff were told, could hardly be experiencing very much more than the minor and passing stresses of adolescence. Even so, as mere youth workers based in an unproven voluntary organisation and using informal and open access approaches, they were certainly not be trusted with the kinds of interventions essential for dealing with mental health problems.

The five-year mental health project which YDT was eventually able to set up in 1980 thus represented a controversial break with conventional mental health practice. Most radically it created a multi-disciplinary staff team made up of a youth worker, a psychiatric social worker and a counsellor. This operated on a dual premise: that youth work values and approaches were essential to welcoming and engaging distressed young people; and that, though still needing to be located in an informal, non-patronising and young person-centred environment, more formal counselling and other skilled therapeutic services then needed to be put on offer.

At the heart of 42nd Street's living history therefore has been, in the words of two of the current workers *'a balanced team of workers producing an inter-penetration of different approaches which are equally respected'*. This commitment has not just meant exploiting the potential of both youth work and therapy as distinctive disciplines. It has also required a sustained and painstaking negotiation of the inevitable dilemmas generated by interweaving two such often divergent and even competing professional ideologies and cultures. Different workers described this as a meeting of *'two irreconcilable models'* and of *'different world views, ideologies'*.

Not surprisingly, such an enterprise has not been without its strains: the last worker quoted regretted, for example, that at times it seemed that within 42nd Street *'there's no base-line understanding from training or a common qualification.*

What's missing is a common agency language'. One long-serving worker on the other hand saw such strains in an entirely positive light, noting that *'42nd Street's external reputation is centred on a commitment to holding a creative tension between youth work and formal therapy'*. This conclusion has had some more objective endorsement – by, for example, the Mental Health Foundation which, in its influential report *Bright Futures*, went so far as to advocate 42nd Street's commitment to this interweaving of formality and informality as a possible model for future practice:

'42nd Street is a voluntary sector project ... providing a range of community-based services for young people who are experiencing a wide range of mental health problems. The project offers individual work in the form of counselling, informal support and befriending relationships. Alongside this they offer an extensive group work programme which includes a weekly drop-in, suicide/self-harm group, and groups for young lesbians, gay men and bisexuals.

'Within its overall brief of meeting the needs of young people within a broad youth work philosophy, the development of distinctive projects has led to a number of important developments ...' [8]

Young people coming to 42nd Street are thus now offered a diverse mix and match of options which take in both informal and quite formal forms of one-to-one contact and structured as well as more open-door and fluid experiences in groups. As a result, according to one worker *'you can see young people moving in and out of roles in different settings – and so see the young person for who they are'*. In addition to meeting differing personal needs, individuals are able to use this range of services for dealing with priorities and concerns as they change over time and also, as one worker put it, for *'addressing different parts of themselves'*:
'A young person coming to 42nd Street can be sat in a counselling room one day exploring feelings about their childhood, and the next day on a minibus to Alton Towers for an activity day with other young people.'

[8] *Bright Futures: Promoting children and young people's mental health*, Mental Health Foundation 1999.

One hospital-based psychotherapist observed that, by offering users the chance to move across the boundaries of such contrasting situations, 42nd Street was arguably recognising the aim of all psychotherapeutic work: '... *the possibility of a young woman moving within 42nd Street from a counselling session to sit on a (staff) recruitment panel to going on a trip to Holland to attending the Resource management committee to attending a policy strategy meeting in London – it may help her make sense of her various "selves" in a very direct-way.*'

Access to this repertoire of methods has other potential pay-offs for young people. While sharpening their capacity to think about and understand their internal world and developmental processes, it also helps, for example, to promote an awareness of the social dimensions of their difficulties. As one worker put it, when applied to experiences of sexual violence: '*Survivors can be presented either with good politics ("you're not on your own") or with good therapy ("we're here to help you look at your feelings") to help them make sense of what is happening to them and move on. Often they are asked to choose between the two– and are then pathologised for making a choice. A mixed social/psychological model at its best can offer both.*'

Or, in the words of a former worker: '*42nd Street offers counselling – one-to-one work which requires young people to identify themselves as needing some help. Its youth work – which doesn't require this kind of self-identification – enables young people to support each other, make friendships.*'

Defining clear and confident professional identities

By '*raising positive challenges for workers about taken-for-granted roles and limits on their work*' (former worker), these daily multi-disciplinary encounters also act as an extra stimulus to staff learning and professional development. Most obviously, they require managers, workers and volunteers to understand – even often to take some personal ownership of – methods which may be unfamiliar and perhaps even threatening. No less important, however, is the expectation built into such an environment that staff can and will articulate what most critically defines and justifies their own primary professional identity and discipline. For, notwithstanding the efforts at integration, these remain as distinctive entities within 42nd Street practice.

'Therapy'

Users' accounts of why they first came to 42nd Street and why they have stayed provide some of the most vivid expositions of 'therapy' in action within the agency. Though usually implicit, they also offer insights into the range of theoretical perspectives and professional training on which this draws:

'It's like a drip ... They're teaching me how to breathe ...'

'In the one-to-one, it's as if they're in your mind. You're telling them ... and they just listen. They don't advise – they ask you what you need... It's okay to cry.'

'Workers get inside you. It's a chance to express yourself. It's okay not to be macho.'

'It means talking about things I've said to no-one – better than bottling things up ... They don't write people off.'

'It's better than bottling things up. It's helped my nightmares.'

'It's helped me sort myself out – not to lose my temper, to speak to my mam.'

'You get one-to-one support. I don't drink as much now.'

'I've been able to talk about my problems. It's not made them go away – I never expected that. They calm me down.'

Workers' more professionalised explanations of the psycho-therapeutic approaches being used, while frequently emphasising *'starting from the young person's own definition of the problem'*, invariably assume *'the use of your therapeutic skills to check things out'* (worker). As we have seen, for one funder this most crucially involved *'providing the right listening ear – without patronising, without pomposity'* while for a worker from a counselling background it included: *'... building up trust, empathy – being very discreet. There has to be real genuineness – something very personal between worker and young person. And an openness of feelings. There are risks to be taken – some real challenges build up.'*

Often drawing on learning from the social work courses many were doing, volunteers added their own supportive reflective clarifications to a discourse on therapy which seemed deeply embedded within 42nd Street's everyday culture.

Nor is this targeted and intensive exploration of how young people are feeling, why they have those feelings and how they might confront and sustain work on damaging emotional and psychological pressures and traumas confined to one-to-one counselling. For one young person for example: *'The suicide and self-harm group is great. I've tried suicide, and thought about it again. The group snapped me out of it. I've not thought about it since – it saved me. I don't know what would have happened.'*

During one staff planning meeting, a worker specifically pressed colleagues to encourage users to take part in an arts event being offered by an external agency because *'the workers there do a lot of self-esteem work'*

The 42nd Street commitment to 'therapy' thus emerges as a coherent and confident component of its professional identity, not only within but also without the organisation. Two referring agencies specifically quoted its reputation for using trained counsellors as a main reason for referring young people to it while funders took it as given that its capacity to go on delivering recognisable therapeutic outcomes to young people must remain a crucial test of its effectiveness – and credibility. This, too, was a key measure for users, as the young person speaking about *One-to-one support – My lifeline* at the start of this chapter, illustrates vividly.

'Youth work'

'The role of youth work values and assumptions remains fundamental... Put at its simplest ... without youth work approaches young people would just not approach the service.' (worker)

'42nd Street has flexible approaches through its youth work, its outreach. It's working with young people where they are – is proactive in going to them.' (funder)

Though, like many other agencies, 42nd Street struggles at times to offer sharply delineated conceptualisations of its youth work approach, these comments capture how central the approach is to the distinctiveness – even, still, the unconventionality – of its style and methodology as a 'mental health agency'. What then, in this context, are the defining characteristics of this method?

One perhaps over-simple answer is that: youth work creates **an environment and an atmosphere which is explicitly young people-friendly:***'42nd Street recognises that where the agency is based is important and that it must not have institutional associations; the name of the agency is crucial; so is what appears on the walls, and how the premises are furnished and decorated ... and how the service is advertised, and how easy it is for young people to make first contact.'* (Worker) Making an almost direct link with the anti-psychiatry climate out of which 42nd Street originally emerged, this same worker added: *'For a mental health agency these ideas in themselves were near revolutionary when compared with psychiatric service waiting rooms and attitudes.'*

Even while highlighting the importance of attractive premises, 42nd Street has also drawn heavily on the **outreach and detached work methods** pioneered by experimental youth work projects in the 1960s and 1970s, including the Youth Development Trust itself. These methods have enabled the agency to extend its geographical reach from the city centre – for example, to Wythenshawe at the extreme southern end of Manchester and into the boroughs of Trafford and Salford. They have also propelled its work directly into other agencies – for example, into offering unfamiliar support to under-paid and often poorly trained staff on the frontline of work with young people in hostels.

The methods of detached youth work have also influenced 42nd Street's consistent use of ***informal group work***. Starting where young people are starting, including their recreational interests, this is often – on users' own evaluation – unashamedly *'easy going, relaxing and an opportunity for a chat.'* Such work particularly embraces forms of activity-based provision which can often at first sight look little different from a conventional adolescent leisure programme. Such programmes, however, are now recognised well beyond 42nd Street as vehicles for effective 'alternative' therapies for dealing with stress and even severe mental health problems.

At 42nd Street informal group work has thus been offered through:

◆ a suicide and self-harm group based on a social action model;

◆ Spice of Life groups for young people, looking at such issues as gender, education and careers;

◆ groups for young women survivors of sexual abuse;

◆ drop-in groups;

◆ creative writing, arts and sports;

◆ trips, residentials and holidays;

◆ a magazine carrying users' articles, poems, drawings and other contributions;

◆ the techniques and remedies of alternative medicines;

◆ involvement in a Campaign against Sexual Abuse rally in London; and

◆ a drama presentation to a Mental Health Foundation Conference.

42nd Street can also be seen to have been deeply marked by the youth work tradition in less pragmatic and more principled ways. For example:

◆ In the context of much mental health treatment which is highly coercive even when notionally voluntary, 42nd Street has been unswerving in its respect for perhaps **the** defining principle of youth work: *young people's right to choose whether or not to get or to stay involved.* In the words of users: *'You please yourself whether you come or not. You please yourself when you come.'*

◆ Unlike their experience in most other youth-serving agencies, at 42nd Street **young people are treated** *as* **young people** rather than as embodiments of labels attached to them by powerful others. Moreover, as we saw from the last chapter, this principle is applied even when the labels include, for example, 'mental patient', 'self-harmer' or 'abuse survivor'.

◆ Within 42nd Street, not just contact but sustained **interaction** *among* **young people is actively sought – indeed proactively promoted**. This is done on the grounds not only that *'it (gives) them some understanding of the wider world'*, but also because: *'... peer support and sharing of life histories and life events all serve to break down the belief of some young people that these things have only happened to them and that therefore they are to blame, they are bad ... It enables them to break down the isolation and fear in their lives.'* (worker)

As a result, as one management member put it: *'The youth work tradition encourages confidence-building because it requires young people to do things together. It's a genuine alternative for some young people to counselling and more formal forms of group work.'*

Users' own testimony repeatedly confirmed such gains. Sample responses included: *'Other people here have the same problems (as me). They help themselves by helping you'*; and *'Other young people at 42nd Street have been through the same things I've been through – so I don't feel they're as serious or peculiar as I thought they were'.*

◆ As it is for youth work generally, tipping balances of power in young people's favour, especially through **user participation**, is seen within 42nd Street as much more than a useful by-product of other activities or as a pragmatic way of achieving other goals. Rather, without denying the complexities and dilemmas of implementing such a commitment (see Chapter 4), it is sought as a desirable end in its own right – indeed as one of the agency's defining features.

Powerful though its impact on 42nd Street has been, this formulation of youth work is seen by some within the agency as now lacking the radical edge which has characterised 42nd Street's wider aspirations and commitments throughout its history. It has been to help re-sharpen that edge that the 'social action' pilot work outlined in the previous chapter is being undertaken – for example, with users who have attempted suicide and who self-harm. The model itself, for example, seeks explicitly to go beyond 'traditional ... participative youth work', with one of 42nd Street's own workers emphasising that *'social action is different from social education'* and another illustrating the difference by outlining a Suicide and Self-Harm Awareness Day run entirely by young people:

'For the first time in 42nd Street's history a whole day was to be young person-led in the fullest sense of the words. Young people from the suicide self-harm group wanted to be heard by a wide audience. They took on all responsibility for deciding when it should happen (during school holidays so under 16s could attend), who they should invite (who they wanted to hear their message and views), and arranging lunch for all participants. They spent a lot of time getting together their own resources and information based on their own experiences which they then displayed on the walls. They also produced a participants' pack with useful contact numbers and a book list.

'The young people involved decided to run the workshops themselves – they wanted people to see that there was more to them than their self-harm. These consisted of a relaxation workshop, an art workshop and a workshop looking at the responses they hoped to get from Accident and Emergency staff. They also did a 'Jerry Springer' kind of drama looking at suicide and self-harm, ending the day with a question and answer session. Approximately thirty participants attended.

'The young people's own evaluation afterwards was very upbeat: "We sat down afterwards for a short chat on the day. We were tired but on a high. There was a sense of achievement in the group. We'd done it and it all went right and we felt we had got our message across to people. This is a rare opportunity for us to get our views across because it was done by us, the people who experience suicide and self-harm in our lives. We could tell people what it is really like for us and what help we really need. All we want is to be listened to and not told who we are and what we need. A little understanding goes a long way."'

More widely, the social action model has provoked a sharp professional debate.[9] This has focused not just on **how** but also on **whether** power can be as fully transferred to young people as social action's stated principles propose, especially when agency and workers are wholly or partially state sponsored. Significantly, within such debates can be detected echoes of older and deeper professional conflicts between the politically oriented forms of community development from which social action sprang and more traditional forms of person-centred youth work.

The adoption of this model of practice is thus likely to pose 42nd Street with a not unfamiliar challenge to its capacity for safeguarding both baby and bath water. Can it embrace the new practice thinking and directions which social action seeks to encourage while preserving the strengths derived over two decades from its embrace of longer established youth work principles and approaches?

'Informal support'

42nd Street's commitment to integrating youth work and formal therapy includes a middle ground – in the form of what the agency calls informal support. This is seen as *'standing equal to and yet distinct from formal counselling'* – but also as *'a key example of therapeutic intervention (which) is one contribution to efforts to provide a clearer theoretical and ideological base for youth work'*. (worker)

---

[9] See *Youth and Policy,* issue numbers 54, 60 and 62.

Like the other core methods in use within 42nd Street, it seeks to empower young people through increased understanding of themselves and their interface with (however defined) their wider community, and of the broader social and political pressures they face. However, it is seen as having some distinctive features:

◆ It takes account of young people's perceptions and expectations of their needs but also of how they might wish to receive 'help' – particularly those who *'come via the mental health system, very withdrawn and with chaotic lives who may not be able to talk through their experiences one-to-one in counselling'.* (worker)

◆ It may take place in a wide range of community-based settings where young people feel comfortable and relaxed and over which they feel they have some control – for example, as one worker noted, *'sitting in Burger King and talking'.*

◆ By legitimising expressions of mutuality and reciprocity between young person and worker, it seeks to break some of the more conventional professional constraints on how the two may relate, what each may disclose – and so how users may be helped.

◆ It not only involves workers from both counselling and youth work backgrounds but overlaps into what volunteers offer, particularly as befrienders – one of whom talked, for example, of *'using my car to move one young person on who's got agoraphobia'.*

Perhaps because it is a hybrid concept which is agency-specific, informal support is not without its critics within 42nd Street. It was, for example, seen by one worker as having *'huge differences of definition within the organisation'* with the result that *'the informal support worker has to develop their own rationale'*; while another worker suggested that *'there's a messiness about what goes on here'*. Thus, for one staff member *'counselling and informal support shade into each other: it's not always clear when not to go into counsellor mode'*; whereas for another *'informal support usually means youth work within 42nd Street'*.

Notwithstanding these reservations and confusions, the very openness of the definition of informal support allows (indeed encourages) workers and perhaps volunteers who see themselves primarily as identified with one of 42nd Street's core practice disciplines to venture into the other. Moreover, they are able to do this by small steps and in an environment which supports the kind of risk-taking involved. This enables informal support to be offered within 42nd Street as a core additional resource to meet the specialist demands of its membership which, despite its emphasis on informality, has been developed as a disciplined method in its own right. Thus, for one worker, while *'stopping short of examining young people's inner processes'*, it required *'exploration of some past associations using the relationship in a very focused reflective way'*. As one volunteer was also very clear, *'I'm not there just to be nice. I also have to set boundaries'*.

Holding tension creatively

Inevitably given its ambition and complexity, by those who must implement it 42nd Street's rhetoric on its multi-disciplinary methodology is not always perfectly delivered nor is it necessarily experienced as entirely liberating. Gaps, inconsistencies and struggles over meanings and interpretations reveal that, on the ground, workers and volunteers are often required to **'hold a creative tension'** (worker) – to distil innovation out of the unresolved and perhaps unresolvable dilemmas produced by, in this case, contrasting professional styles and cultures in criss-crossing orbits.

These tensions show themselves in a number of ways.

A hierarchy of disciplines?

Within any multi-disciplinary team, prior professional socialisation has usually done its job too well for some assumptions about methodological hierarchies not to surface. These are as likely to reflect subjective perceptions of what is going on at least as much as the objective reality. As one worker from a youth work background noted, such perceptions may well anyway have antecedents well beyond an individual agency and its history. For example: *'The youth work model hasn't been strong enough for a mental health service. It's not well articulated, it's underdeveloped. There's been a lack of training, especially for intensive sustained one-to-one relationships ... Youth workers have to end up saying: "we can't work with this".'*

Even a relatively open and reflective milieu like 42nd Street shows the effects of such 'readings'. The perceived lack of focus of informal support, for example, results in some workers seeing it as in effect a sub-category of, and therefore as of lower status than, both counselling and youth work. Perhaps even more significant, 42nd Street's core commitment to achieving 'therapeutic' outcomes leads some, both within and without, to rank counselling as the method which ultimately delivers the agency's goods.

One current worker's view, for example, was that *'there's a hierarchy of disciplines here – and it's not just perceived. We're now a counselling organisation. This can be competitive'.* Even in retrospect, a former worker concluded that *'the culture here seems to put counselling at the top, informal support at the bottom'.* And a referring agency made clear that: *'We send our people to 42nd Street because they have professionally qualified counsellors who do more than we do and sit and talk to young people just because they're down. They make confidential counselling relationships with them.'*

Workers: Retaining professional identities

Where (even implicitly) this kind of hierarchy of methodologies is felt to operate it seemingly downgrades one professional discipline. This may mean that those identifying with this feel de-skilled even perhaps to the point where they question whether their own approaches are valid and still worth offering. One 42nd Street worker, for example, wondered: *'Is the youth worker clever enough to be here – in comparison to the counsellor?'* Another, whose identity was first as a youth worker, concluded: *'I felt like I was being asked to be a counsellor by becoming an informal support worker.'* A former worker asked: *'Who are your peers at 42nd Street? Counsellors? Youth workers? Psychotherapists?'*; while another confessed: *'I wouldn't want to come back. I feel much more effective now – I can operate as I feel I need to. The multi-disciplinary context ... can weaken professional identities.'*

Clearly these reactions are more than balanced by the many other perceptions which stressed the stimulus injected by 42nd Street's multi-disciplinary structure and processes to fresh and open-minded thinking about other forms of analysis and approach. They do nonetheless demonstrate some potentially inhibiting (even if unintended) consequences for some of the practitioners involved in the multi-disciplinary model.

Young people: Negotiating boundaries

For some workers – though not usually, it seemed, for volunteers – the very fluidity of multi-disciplinary working could also strain important professional boundaries with users. This was then seen as posing a risk to some of the young people choosing to come to an agency like 42nd Street who might be unsure of their social skills or were scarred still by previous experiences of adult inconsistency.

Different workers focused such dilemmas in different ways:
'The work can be experienced very conflictually by young people and workers. The worker is setting boundaries for the young person in the counselling relationship – and then is going with them to Alton Towers. Workers are asked to share different versions of themselves. And there are conflicts for young people too.'

'Young people get access to less therapeutically defined encounters and relationships – the members meeting, holidays, the drop-in. This can run against some counsellors' perspectives.'

'The counsellor has to reveal bits of themselves which they aren't normally expected to do. It breaks down barriers – but sometimes confuses the boundaries needed for the counselling relationship.'

Holding together

Such doubts do of course need to be set in the context of the very substantial gains which flow, directly and indirectly, from 42nd Street's multi-disciplinary 'menu'. Starting from a shared, explicit and comprehensive assessment protocol, for young people this opens up rare outlets for some safe 'rehearsal' of new roles and for their negotiation of a range of unfamiliar and sometimes testing situations. Many are then able to explore and try out different (and often, for them, more affirming) 'selves', in the process discovering blocked or unknown possibilities and talents. For workers and volunteers, multi-disciplinary practice provides (again a, still, rare) chance to move towards that elusive goal – a holistic service. By demanding on-going clarification for colleagues of one's own specialist skills while simultaneously requiring a search to understand **their** analyses and expertise, it keeps workers on their toes and so acts as an in-built counter to complacency and professional stagnation.

Here again, the benefits are not, of course, guaranteed. A multi-disciplinary structure and approach has to be **resourced**, particularly to avoid the lowest common denominator risk of staff simply ending up as jills and jacks of all trades. It has to be **managed** – and managed in ways which both set clear boundaries and liberate rather than stifle its potential creativity (see Chapter 6). Such management needs to include adequate and appropriate **supervision** – which in 42nd Street includes both regular internal supervision and extensive forms of external casework consultancy. And space needs to be found for teams and groups (small and large, on-going and short-term) actually to operationalise the **multi-**disciplinary nature of the work.

Ultimately, however, the justification is clear. By holding hard to its belief in multi-disciplinary practice within one specialist youth-serving agency, 42nd Street has provided evidence of the advantages of tailor-making practice for young people who, precisely because of their confusion and distress, need the chance to choose and the time to grow into the best form of 'treatment' **for them**.

Chapter 4: Participation

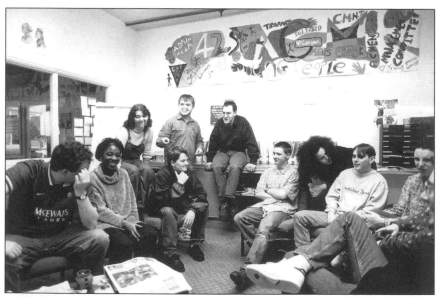

The SmithKline Beecham Impact Award Group meet to plan their presentations.

Chapter 4: Participation

Participation as panacea?

Commitments to participation have appeared regularly in work with young people. As we saw in the last chapter, they have been particularly important to the youth work tradition which has so influenced 42nd Street. During the 1990s, the rhetoric of participation was seized on, too, by state policy makers looking for more sophisticated techniques for managing an increasingly alienated adolescent age group.

Yet, as 42nd Street would be the first to acknowledge, getting beyond tokenism – securing young people's authentic and sustained contributions to consultative and decision-making mechanisms and even perhaps to actual service delivery – is a highly complex process. Here above all it is essential to start where they are, to operate on their ground, move at their pace, continue to recognise them as individuals with often pressing personal needs. Where, driven by a liberal enthusiasm to 'do the right thing', these crucial ground rules are ignored, the results can be counter-productive. As one group of researchers found: *'Poor participatory mechanisms are very effective in training young people to become non-participants.'* [10]

The reasons for such realism are not hard to find:

◆ Because of their lack of years, to say nothing of the stigmatised definitions of youth itself, most young people are likely to have been treated for much of their lives as unreliable and untrustworthy and so as incapable of carrying responsibility.

◆ They are likely therefore to have had few opportunities, through practice and

[10] Hugh Matthews, Melanie Limb, Lisa Harrison and Mark Taylor, 'Local Places and the Political Engagement of Young People, *Youth & Policy*, No. 62, pp.16–30.

experience, of gaining the confidence needed to take the risks **for them** of commitment to participatory activities. Nor will they have had chance to develop much personal ownership of the skills and knowledge required, especially for working the formal committee-type machinery on which adults so often insist. Often, therefore, the only young people to take the participatory bait are a self-selected elite with little accountability to or credibility with their notional 'constituency'.

◆ Even where they are consulted, young people's views and suggestions are readily ignored or their priorities reinterpreted to satisfy adult expectations. Thus, while research shows that for young people jobs, leisure outlets and less hostile community and police attitudes are the priorities, service providers are still most likely to advocate vocational training and community safety.[11] Unsurprisingly, young people then end up distrusting adult efforts to get them to participate.

For many of the young people being targeted by 42nd Street, these wider deficits will have been exacerbated by damaging life experiences. As one referring agency explained: *'Our young people are far less secure, less well educated. They often come from disabling backgrounds and have never been asked their opinion on anything or to make a decision on important aspects of their lives. They've been further disabled by the services they've been in contact with.'*

Therapy for self-empowerment

Despite having often to learn and re-learn these lessons through hard experience, 42nd Street's commitment to a user voice and user input has been maintained since its earliest days. Underpinning it has been, in the words of one worker: *'... a recognition of (young people's) wealth of experience and knowledge in dealing with mental health, mental illness, stress, suicide and self-harm and depression etc. (Because) their experiences are valid ... we need to know from them what works and*

---

[11] *Including Young People in Urban Regeneration,* Joseph Rowntree Foundation, September 1998.

what doesn't ... to acknowledge that they were surviving long before the worker came along and will continue to survive long after the worker has moved on.'

Flowing from such a premise has been a bedrock commitment to young people's empowerment within the primary methodologies used within 42nd Street – that is, within its counselling relationships, its youth work and social action programmes and its provision of informal support (see Chapter 3). While offering both resources and challenge, these aim to develop young people's motivations and capacities for acting autonomously and for taking maximum control of their own lives. As one external agency explained: *'Some of the young people we refer come back with a new confidence, feeling worth something and valued ... That's empowered them.'*

These principles are most conventionally embodied in procedures on, for example, non-disclosure of information without the young person's permission and, as far as possible, expectations that **they** will make the necessary contacts with other agencies. However, as young people take on their individual challenges, the help they give each other through formal and informal forms of group work and more casual social interaction is also seen as an expression of the agency's participation ethic.

Participation in policy making and decision-making

If empowerment does not take place here, within the everyday therapeutic interactions of an agency like 42nd Street, attempts elsewhere in the organisation to reorder power relationships are unlikely to have much meaning. Within its governance and constitutional arrangements this, however, is also an explicit, and ambitious, aspiration. The goal is not the well-intentioned but ultimately self-deluding one of transferring to young people indiscriminate segments of the power necessarily exercised by workers, managers, Resources Management Committee (RMC) members and funders as part of their given roles. As one group of workers pointed out: *'42nd Street might be trying to be a young person-centred organisation. It is not young people led.'*

Other limits to the power and responsibility users can carry are also acknowledged, particularly to avoid setting them up to fail. For example, it is recognised that:

◆ goals need to be agreed with which **they** identify and which it is feasible for them to pursue;

◆ roles and tasks need to be defined which take into account their personal starting points of confidence, motivation and skill; and

◆ if young people are to take these on, sometimes quite lengthy processes have to be worked through which require ongoing (and usually labour-intensive) support and training.

However, within 42nd Street these parameters are not seen primarily as constraints on users, nor are they treated as immutable. Rather, their enunciation – including, in appropriate language, to young people – is used positively. Their main aim is to delineate by mutual agreement a wide range of safe and supported areas of the agency's practice in which young people can, with increasing confidence, exercise the forms of influence and control which are appropriately theirs. To clarify these structural roles within the organisation as well as to boost their *'sense of belonging'* (worker), 42nd Street's users have now become members rather than the consumers described in the publications of the 1980s.

Constitutionally and indeed politically, these commitments have come to be expressed in a number of concrete ways, some of which are underpinned materially through the payment of expenses to the young people who take part.

◆ Members are encouraged to attend meetings of the RMC which are open meetings. As a group they have control over three voting places. They also take part as of right in the work of subcommittees, working parties, conference presentations, 'away days' and similar forums.

◆ Decisions and recommendations from the monthly members' meeting are formally fed into RMC business by members, not all of whom have to be the named representatives. The need for RMC responses to these is taken as read.

◆ Over a number of years, members have made prominent and sometimes critical inputs into the organisation's Annual General Meetings.

◆ With preparation and support, members organise their own recruitment panels for all fieldwork posts and have one vote in the final decision-making process.

◆ Members are routinely involved in lobbying delegations to funders.

◆ Members are encouraged and supported to speak at conferences.

◆ Members are given the choice to deal with media requests for comment and contributions.

As we shall see later, implementing these more formalised forms of participation carries its own dilemmas and tensions. Nonetheless, they too represent crucial expressions, in policy and practice, of 42nd Street's commitment to young people's empowerment.

Developing a culture of empowerment

This commitment does not stop here, however. It assumes, too, what might be called a **culture** of empowerment whose defining characteristics include:

◆ A recognition of young people's claims on power and influence which permeates all the agency's interactions and activities and has touched many users in personal ways. As one worker expressed it: *'Can you work in 42nd Street with young people and never do a piece of participation work?'*

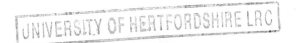

◆ An acceptance therefore that, in all their encounters with users, all those involved in the organisation need self-consciously at the very least to avoid **dis**empowering them and, as far as possible, proactively to encourage and nurture – to **embrace** – empowering interventions and relationships.

◆ As defined by one worker, such a culture, is seen as part of a wider fluidity which ensures that *'participation ... does not become stagnant'*. It also assumes the need to *'move from asking young people to be involved in projects that are good politically for 42nd Street or ... in work that a worker thinks would be useful ... to young people being proactive in having their needs met'*.

◆ It assumes, too, that the focus of user participation goes beyond concerns and issues internal to 42nd Street to include inputs into external policy developments and events crucial to users' interests.

A minority of workers were not wholly convinced that 42nd Street was *'working collectively enough with young people'* (worker) to capitalise on their common experiences and shared identities. One for example quoted: *'(Some) groups tend to look internally and work on things like assertiveness. Perhaps they should give more attention to the young people's collective voices against homophobia or racism.'*

Another raised a similar point specifically in relation to mental health issues:
'Our help for young people to participate in direct action against the mental health system is pretty token. For example, we have no contacts with the organisations campaigning against ECT.'

Other evidence points strongly to the conclusion emphasised by another worker that: *'... participation is (treated as) political ... because ... (it) gives young people a chance to glimpse and ultimately grasp their own power ... to see that they are not alone in attempting to bring change in their own lives ... that change is possible.'*

This worker added: *'Without young people's voices where would 42nd Street be? In all my contacts with external agencies it is young people's voices and experiences they want to hear.'*

Even more convincing was the description of where the experience of participation had led him and others offered by one user writing in the 1999 42nd Street Annual Report: *'It is sometimes said that one opportunity is a doorway to another. In our experience of the participation work at 42nd Street, this is most certainly true. It all really started when we were taking part in the Mental Health Foundation inquiry ... Because of (our) presentation (we were invited) to the House of Lords for the launch of the findings of the inquiry ... We were soon recognised as "the young people from 42nd Street" ... Although we felt like token youths at the beginning of the evening, our discussions ... demonstrated that we think very deeply about mental health issues and ... have a lot to contribute ... We try to keep constantly in mind that we want to make a positive difference to mental health services in this country ...'*

Another vivid example of users applying this *'wider view of themselves as active citizens'* (worker) emerged from the process leading up to their involvement in the Trafalgar Square child sexual abuse rally in September 1999 at which 42nd Street members spoke from the platform. As described by one worker: *'This was a request put forward by a young person and picked up by other users ... They were able to take part in the rally and have a clear understanding of why they were there, that this was an issue which affected them personally and that they had a right to say something about it – they needed to be listened to.'*

A range of other examples illustrates this broader culture of empowerment at work within and beyond 42nd Street

◆ Part-funded by 42nd Street, in 1999 two 42nd Street members went as UK representatives to a United Nations conference on the environment and mental health held in Hawaii.

◆ In 1999 users helped conceive, plan and carry through a visit to Holland and in 2000 to Slovenia. The latter involved visits to youth and social work projects.

◆ Over a number of years, users have made substantial planned inputs to public conferences on suicide and self-harm. They have also taken the initiative to organise a suicide and self-harm 'awareness day' in April 2000, aimed at workers and young people (see Chapter 3).

◆ As an assertion of their sense of ownership of the organisation, young women users designed their own banner which they then unfurled at the 1999 AGM.

◆ Writing as users of 42nd Street, members have published a number of articles on mental health issues and services.

◆ With support from within 42nd Street, users have struggled to make good use of both the local and national media, working hard to avoid the exploitation of their personal experiences while at the same time sharing these on occasion as a way of increasing public understanding of what it is like to be young and under stress.

42nd Street participatory realities – and tensions

Here again, however, reality – rarely if ever as clear-cut or as straightforward as such descriptions suggest – contains a number of tensions, contradictions and possible gaps.

Age groups

Lowering its age limit to 14 and establishing a specific Children and Young People's Team have represented major developments for 42nd Street. In particular these have offered greater accessibility for, and more proactive preventive work with, younger people, resulting by May 2000 in a surge of over 50 per cent of all new referrals falling within the 14 to 18-year-old age range.

At the same time it has posed new questions, not about whether younger users can participate, but about how their involvement can be nurtured and how this can be done alongside inputs by users 10 or more years older than them and with some very different life experiences. This tension was initially reflected, for example, in the women's drop-in group. At one stage older members withdrew from this, complaining that it had become too much like a youth club. However, as more 14 to 18-year-olds became assimilated more widely into the agency, their evaluations changed – for example:

'(It's) good. People of different ages act different. You get to see what they're like.'

'There's no good and bad. We treat each other the same.'

The gap – including the participation gap – can clearly be bridged.

Specialist or generalist?

As we have seen, a core principle of 42nd Street's approach is that *'participation touches all aspects of our work (and so) cannot be pigeonholed into one project'* (worker). At the same time it has for a number of years committed 10 worker hours weekly to participation work plus some volunteer time and has now established two specialist part-time participation posts providing 28 worker hours a week.

Such dual approaches, however, invariably carry a significant risk. On the one hand, they may encourage 'generalist' workers to relax on the premise that the 'real' participation work is being done by the specialists. Meanwhile, the specialists may build up relationships, expertise and a body of knowledge which (albeit unintentionally) reduce or block the generalists' access to this area of practice.

Open or exclusive?

Notwithstanding a strong supportive rhetoric about open access to the agency's participative processes and machinery, a further risk is that drift will occur towards exclusivity and elitism. Here too the contradiction is deeply built in. On the one hand, for youth participation to work, as well as to produce identifiable practical gains, it must be fun and provide satisfying personal relationships (especially with other young people but also with adults). It must also enable those taking part to acquire new skills and insights which then become the building blocks for new self-insights and a new self-confidence.

However, the more such goals are achieved and their rewards experienced personally, the more tempting it is for those involved to turn in on themselves. Again unintentionally, they may then make entry difficult for those who are outside the core group and who have not yet developed the same basic competence and assurance. One former 42nd Street worker, for example, concluded that *'we always seemed to be going back to the same small group – to the same people to represent young people.'* According to one RMC member, a *'participation group seems to be developing which is quite small in relation to the whole membership. How accessible is this group? How far is this work percolating through the whole organisation? How accountable are they?'* It was this committee member, too, who pondered: *'I'm not always clear where young women's voices are in these discussions.'*

Critical or tamed?

Not unrelated is the risk of drawing such activist users so deeply into an organisation's given dominant ideas and ways of working that the critical perspectives which make their contributions distinctive become blunted and are even perhaps lost altogether. One RMC member, reflecting on the 42nd Street participation processes, asked: *'How far do we incorporate our young people? They often seem incredibly polite participants! For example, on the issues being raised, how far have they really affected our policy and direction, I wonder?'*

Member power, worker power – and agency control?

While the *StreetCred?* consultations were taking place some acrimonious debate occurred within 42nd Street on the appearance in one of the user areas of a graffiti board containing what some saw as offensive material and a women's group display containing some anti-male slogans. On one side were those who argued that both innovations were no more than expressions of members' views which, because they stayed within the 42nd Street ground rules, were legitimate. Others, however, suggested that the displays were more worker than member inspired.

The substantive issues under scrutiny were (appropriately) about the content of the displays (see, for example, Chapter 5) and led to vigorous discussion in both the worker team and among users, particularly in members' meetings. A meeting with men and women members set up to promote discussion and communication between them contributed eventually to a positive process for users negotiating their shared use and membership of 42nd Street. However, embedded within these debates, too, was an ambiguity – not of course at all special to 42nd Street – about how to define the boundary between member and worker power and, perhaps even more crucial, who had the greatest leverage for deciding this.

Another case study of similarly contradictory signals was 42nd Street's first residential trip for members outside the UK: a five-day visit to Amsterdam. With young people taking responsibility for deciding on everything from the preferred destination, fundraising and ground rules through to practicalities like accommodation and flights, here too the indistinct lines between support and (even unintentional) control needed constantly to be monitored. The trip also provoked more principled debates within the staff team and the RMC. Was a holiday experience sufficient justification or should it contain an explicit educational component? And why Amsterdam, with its known (and stereotyped) liberal drugs policy? Yet for the young people – many going abroad for the first time – the whole point was that they were carrying the responsibility personally and as a group and what is more in a strange and challenging environment.

As 42nd Street proceeds with is attempts to integrate a social action model into its practice, this challenge may move from the pragmatic to the more fundamentally principled. For, if social action stands for anything, it is that, in becoming empowered, young people should not be confined within the given organisational parameters of a particular agency. Rather, it is for them to determine the basic structures in which their impact on decision-making is to be achieved. Even allowing for the openness and flexibility of 42nd Street's participative mechanisms and processes and the undoubted influence of users on these so far, this would seem to require some substantial steps beyond where it has reached so far.

Participation or efficiency?

Much more explicit – indeed, often, it seemed, anguished – was a concurrent dialogue within 42nd Street on members' participation in the RMC. As we have seen, the mechanisms and procedures here are clearly established and well used. Brief observation suggested, too, that in practice genuine opportunities exist for users to be involved and their inputs treated seriously. Moreover, with discussion taking place in an open circle rather than behind formal tables, and earnestness being tempered by an egalitarian and sometimes self-deprecating humour, the overall style of these exchanges seemed also to support young people's participation.

However, the unintended effects of such openness also raise a number of questions:

◆ How can member representation get beyond tokenism when effective participation in RMC business often requires substantial and sophisticated technical information and knowledge, including about national policies, which users will at the very least need time (and the motivation) to acquire?

◆ What is the appropriate balance between, on the one hand, ensuring that members' views influence RMC thinking and decisions and, on the other, providing the committee with the time it needs to take and follow up often complex decisions across a wide range of agenda items?

◆ Given that most RMC lay members can offer only limited time to their RMC work, how can efficient conduct of RMC business be combined with a (time-consuming) open-door policy for users to attend and contribute? (This dilemma was fleetingly but pointedly acknowledged at the start of one RMC meeting when a worker reminded the 14 young people present that the main business of the meeting required RMC members to fulfil their legal and other responsibilities to 42nd Street.)

What these questions highlight is that, in pursuing such participation, clarity about **primary** purposes is vital. Thus, though involvement in the work of a body such as the 42ⁿᵈ Street RMC may be a valuable vehicle for young people's development as participators, ultimately this is not the committee's raison d'être. Rather, it exists to agree agency policy and provide the organisation with strategic management. As one administrative worker acknowledged: *'We're at a crossroads with participation – especially in relation to the RMC now there's mass take-up. There are strains over participation versus efficiency and also some value conflicts. Especially now because of our size – staff turnover, relations with outside bodies, etc. – there's lots of business. The emphasis now is on professionalism and efficiency – it's a different culture.'*

From participation to therapy – and beyond

Not everyone associated with 42ⁿᵈ Street judges its energetic pursuit of user participation as guaranteeing therapeutic gains for young people. Some of these doubts reflect wider questions (raised in Chapter 3) about maintaining appropriate boundaries as a young person moves (perhaps with the same worker in support) from, say, one-to-one work to a committee role or conference present-ation. One worker, for example, suggested that *'young people are in and out of their different selves – from the vulnerability and the pain of a counselling situation to the empowerment of a part in the RMC'.* Another questioned *'whether it's always therapeutic to participate – whether it's always in young people's best interests. Might we sometimes be setting them up to fail again?'* And a former worker worried that *'as young people (especially perhaps young women) developed their participation skills, these might be masking their psychological and mental health needs ... How far did the work on participation overpower their individual needs?'*

Again, however, though important for keeping the debate open and well fuelled, these are undoubtedly minority voices. The broad consensus within 42ⁿᵈ Street is clearly that, in addition to collective political gains, active **and appropriate** roles in decision-making and in delivering a service can nudge on a young person's personal development in highly significant ways. They can increase confidence; broaden horizons; extend social contacts; refine social skills (not least for dealing with adults in authority and in public arenas); confirm the validity of personal experience and deepen understandings of personal problems by placing them in broader contexts; and lead to a discovery of talents which have been buried, denied – or never previously glimpsed. Indeed, *'because of the change it can bring in young people's ... sense of self'* (worker), 'participation' – the opportunity to exercise responsibility and power – is widely seen as making substantial and positive mental health contributions to young lives which to that point have often been overwhelmed by exclusion and powerlessness.

Here, it would seem, a circle is completed, with the therapeutic benefits produced for 42nd Street's users emerging as a – perhaps the – justification for giving participation such high priority. Certainly, within 42nd Street, young people's often all but uncritical evaluation of their participation experiences can contrast sharply with the anguishing of some of the adults over its pros and cons.

This conclusion is thrown into special relief when seen against a backdrop of a mental health services tradition which (to put it at its most generous) has shown little enthusiasm for 'power-to-the-patient' strategies. Some of these attitudes may now be shifting as funders insist on user consultation and on evaluation which at least takes into account users' experiences. What these seemingly flavour-of-the-month endorsements often fail to do, however, is to consider how the given professional and bureaucratic power balances within user-provider relationships – and above all the deeply ingrained habit of 'doing to' patients – might substantively even if only partially be reconstituted.

In retrospect it is possible to discern that – slowly, with some deliberation, often drawing heavily on the wisdom of hindsight following stumbles or even failures – 42nd Street has over its 20-year history been engaged in developing just such a participation project. In the process, some entrenched 'helping' boundaries have been both clarified and redrawn and some conventional roles and relationships redefined. As a result, young people – including those known to others as 'mentally ill' – have asserted their opinions and their rights and taken on responsibilities in ways which neither they nor the agency had initially thought was within their remit – or their capability.

Chapter 5: Equal opportunities

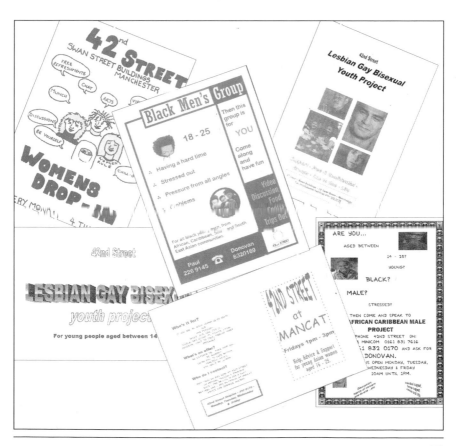

Chapter 5: Equal opportunities

What kind of equal opportunities?

Few self-respecting 'helping' organisations entered the 21st century without declaring their equal opportunities credentials. Indeed, some seemed to be suggesting that they had reached such a state of grace that all who crossed their threshold were guaranteed unimpeded access and unblemished non-prejudicial treatment. Apparently untouched by the 'isms, which, like a resort's name through a stick of rock, run inextricably through British society, all complexity and contradiction had, they implied, been dissipated. The words having been enunciated, the equality deed was done.

Usually implicit in such simplistic positions was an equally simplistic analysis of the problems to be tackled. As one experienced 42nd Street volunteer expressed it: *'It was usually assumed in other agencies I've worked in that "prejudice" is the problem'* – that is, that all will be well if one inappropriate or unhelpful staff or user attitude after another is adjusted or eliminated. As if to endorse this, throughout the period the *StreetCred?* project was under way, large public bodies continued to insist that, to deal with their discriminatory practices, all they needed to do was to root out a few bad apples. Thus the Metropolitan Police Force remained unbending in its denials that its investigations of Stephen Lawrence's murder had in any way been touched by institutional racism. Teachers' organisations have reacted with similar disbelief to suggestions that institutional racism was common in schools.

Clearly, following through the logic of more institutionally focused definitions of oppression means moving beyond a concern simply with discrete personal experiences and serial one-to-one exchanges. It requires, too, confronting the possibility that whole groups or categories of people may be encountering systematic discrimination. As such responses usually have deep historical and organisational roots, this may then demand that structures and procedures be changed or at least that the worst effects of their routine ways of operating be ameliorated. In turn, this may call for a direct challenge to the way power is distributed and used, not only within the organisation itself but in society more widely.

Making the rhetoric real

From its inception, 42nd Street took up a clear and uncompromising stance on equal opportunities. It was after all set up to cater for individuals and groups – most obviously young people and 'the mentally ill' – for whom access to a wide range of crucial resources, acceptance and equity of treatment were often especially elusive. Its reframed statement of intent in 1997 stressed that *'oppression and discrimination exist in our society and affects us in many ways, especially in relation to gender, race, disability and sexual preference'*. For the volunteer quoted above, some elements of 42nd Street's stance on equal opportunities were in 1999 still *'unusual and unexpected'* – particularly this emphasis on young people's *'different identities (and) the extra problems groups take on because of their sexuality, for example'*.

By the mid 1990s, progress was being recorded in *'addressing issues which affect all groups of people who experience oppression in this society'*.

◆ Appropriate forms of training and outreach for excluded constituencies had been provided, including through collaborative work with other agencies.

◆ Steps had been taken to recruit Black workers (including volunteers) with (by 1996) extra funding having been gained specifically for work with Black young men and by 2000 for work with Black young women.

◆ Following a move to new premises, access for disabled young people had improved, new plans were being laid to engage 'neglected' groups by producing publicity materials in Braille and on tape, installing an induction loop and ensuring staff used the minicom effectively. By 1999, specific steps had been taken in collaboration with an outside agency to open up the resource more effectively to young people with hearing impairments and to raise additional funds for work with disabled young people generally.

◆ Since 42nd Street's earliest days when young men had dominated the drop-in and other more social groups, work with young women had been given a high priority. Specialist women's counselling posts had been created and regular women's groups established until, the 1995 annual report noted, young women came to outnumber young men.

◆ Partly in response to this but more specifically to mounting national concerns about high suicide and self-harm rates among young men, a young men's project post was created in 1994 to ensure that the needs of young men were not marginalised or overlooked within the project.

◆ New groups had been started, some targeted at the 'double-disadvantaged' – for example, Black women and disabled young men.

◆ Recognising the specific stresses experienced by some lesbians, gay young men and bisexuals, by 1995 a specialist lesbian, gay and bisexual project had been established employing a part-time lesbian worker and a part-time gay man worker.

Relative to 42nd Street's own past performance and especially to what was on offer in many other agencies, a range of perceptions confirmed the impact of these developments:

'Young Black people seem more comfortable at 42nd Street.' (referring agency)

'Black young people have an easier time at 42nd Street. There are some role models for Black young men – it's rare to find proactive non-white workers for that age group in Manchester.' (referring agency)

'42nd Street seems to have got it as good as it can get. There doesn't seem to be any judgment because of sexuality ...' (referring agency)

'It certainly seems to have picked up strongly on sexuality.' (funder)

'For many people 42nd Street seems to be characterised as working with gay, lesbian and bisexual young people, with young people who self-harm, with Black young people. It's perceived largely in relation to those kinds of issues.' (former worker)

Other contributions suggested further that some of the core equal opportunities tenets were also embedding themselves in the agency's everyday culture:

'The staff's acceptance of someone being gay made it easier for me to come out.' (user)

'If there are homophobic incidents, the staff always find out and get people to talk to each other. They deal with it brilliantly.' (user)

'I was nervous when I first went into the (mainly white) drop-in. Would they accept me as new and Black? In the end my colour didn't matter – it was just that I was new. There weren't even slip-of-the-tongue comments.' (volunteer)

'It's not just platitude, a fake, patronising – not even all that vociferous, ideological do-gooding you find in other organisations. It has a genuineness, a reality.' (volunteer)

'It's a real commitment. It assimilates workers into the agency culture.' (admin worker)

'I've never really registered the positive statements. It seems integral therefore taken-for-granted. I pick it up accidentally.' (funder)

In the context of discussion of other matters, one funder described 42nd Street as generally *'unjudgmental'*. Specifically in relation to its work with gay, lesbian and bisexual young people, a referring agency saw it as *'avoiding stigma'* . More than one of these external agencies also commented approvingly on its offer to users to say whether they wish to see a male or female counsellor.

The same principles often expressed themselves in taken-for-granted ways in searching team discussions – for example, on whether responses to a particular male user might need to be 'gendered' and how this could be achieved within a mainly female worker team. They were reflected, too, in a similarly consensual debate – involving workers, RMC members, volunteers and users – on how to ensure that applying the legislation on the declaration of offences did not discriminate against gay men applying to work at 42nd Street.

Limitations and gaps

None of this means, of course, that 42nd Street as an organisation or – regardless of their own ethnicity, gender, sexual orientation or disability – the individuals operating within it have been immune from discriminatory infections. Rather, in complex interaction over the years of its development, all have had to learn and act their way out of some oppressive ways of thinking and practising. As far back as 1986, a developmental study on the agency, *Principles into Practice*, openly faced the fact that at that stage *'significantly fewer young women than young men have found 42nd Street's service accessible'*. Even more striking, the report had nothing at all to say on the other oppressed groups whose use of 42nd Street (or lack of it) so preoccupied contributors to the *StreetCred?* consultations.[12]

Moreover, in 42nd Street no less than in any other agency even when on some issues the rhetoric is strong, it can stubbornly refuse to come together with the reality. Even in mid-1999, for example, wheelchair-users' restricted physical access to the 42nd Street building continued to grab time at both users' and RMC meetings. Despite the development of joint working with some outside agencies, concerns were still being expressed in more than one group discussion about disproportionately low levels of use by Black and Asian young people.

Some of the unease over the application of equal opportunities commitments went deeper, touching on underlying, even principled, limitations. One worker,

---

[12] Aileen McDermott, *Principles into Practice*, 42nd Street, 1986.

for example, suggested that 42nd Street was made up of *'a very educated workforce who can talk the talk on these matters even when not all that much is happening'*. This forthrightness prompted a Black colleague to comment: *'I don't really like to say it but we're still very much a white middle-class counselling agency'* while another worker chose to put the emphasis on 42nd Street as *'a white middle-class male agency'*.

For a few, limited consciousness and analysis meant that the potential of class identity for collective action had remained under-exploited. As we saw in Chapters 3 and 4, an article of faith for 42nd Street is that young people gain motivation and increased capacity for action through strengthened images of, and belief in, themselves as young women, young Black people, young disabled people, young gays, lesbians or bisexuals. Much less apparent were emphases on young people's experiences of, and often sharp insights into, an economic system which repeatedly leaves them poor, highly marginal to the labour market, exploited when they are employed and constantly subject to crude forms of labour discipline when they seek income support.

Dilemmas and contradictions

Such reservations and gaps ultimately emerge as footnotes to a high level of consciousness of equal opportunities issues and concerns about discrimination and oppression. Beyond these, however, the 42nd Street experience demonstrates dilemmas which do seem inherent to practice and policy-making in this area.

Treating everyone the same – or as different?

During the consultations one example of such contradictory pressures was exposed by the working definitions of equal opportunities being used. Thus, while one user emphasised that *'everyone here gets treated the same'*, what was important for one worker was that *'people are treated differently – according to their age or gender for example. Each one needs specific work. It's not just an equal service – to guarantee accessibility, some require more equality than others.'*

The first of these comments came from a young woman seeking to express her approval of 42nd Street's efforts not to pre-judge her merely because she had a psychiatric diagnosis or had self-harmed. The way the organisation had received her, she seemed to be suggesting, had connected most directly to her 'ordinariness'. This contrasted with many previous (especially professional) encounters which, homing in on those experiences and characteristics which highlighted her 'deviance', added to her sense of isolation and even her exclusion from much of the human race.

Yet, as the second statement implies, 'treating everyone the same' carries the risk that an equal opportunities vision will become clouded or even narrowed by a colour or gender blindness or by their discriminatory equivalences experienced by other unpopular and oppressed groups. To be sharp and relevant, this vision requires a recognition that, in our competitive society's race for the good life, entry points are **not** the same for everyone or for the groups with which they identify most strongly. Undifferentiated treatment, individual by individual, will therefore not necessarily realise the vision. As one worker warned: *'You can't just say: here we are, come and use us. Some attitudes are just too entrenched – institutional racism, attitudes to disability.'*

Traditional pluralist Britain does not always take kindly to this kind of interpretation of equal opportunities since it demands that organisational policies and practices be stretched well beyond the much vaunted virtue of tolerating what is different or unusual. When stripped down, this can emerge as a (rather patronising) concession which in effect argues: Even though certain individuals, certain identities, certain cultures deviate from an array of not-to-be-questioned dominant and potentially oppressive norms, we will generously accord them the marginal status of 'okay really'.

By contrast, the more encompassing notion of access and treatment which underpins 42nd Street's struggle towards equal opportunities requires that such diversity is positively and actively **embraced** and indeed **celebrated**. In this way sharp variations from established and traditional ideas, beliefs and practices, in being acknowledged as legitimate and mainstream, are seen as valuable in their own right – and so as extending and deepening the pluralism on which British society so prides itself.

Embracing difference – or neutralising distinctiveness?

Even this movement from tolerance to the active celebration of difference and diversity is not without its contradictory twists, however. Within 42nd Street these show themselves in at least two ways.

At the level of daily action, they are prompted firstly by its decision to **name** some posts and projects as supports for key identity groups using the agency – to, for example, employ specialist workers with Black young men, with young lesbians and with gay men – which have developed significant profiles. The argument here is that, within an organisation whose brief is wide and generalist, fulfilling the commitment to meeting excluded or poorly represented interests needs some investment of substantial and focused resources. How better to do this than by delegating some of it to people who are *'likeminded with the users'* (volunteer) – who *'share their personal experiences'* (volunteer)? Such responses not only appeal to certain funders and have the potential for drawing on likeminded support from young people's own peers. They also fit a key common assumption of many of those involved in 'identity politics': that, ultimately, to understand one you have to be one.

As some of the quotations included earlier in this chapter show, support for such a policy is confirmed by the testimony of users and referring agencies. Yet it also contains dilemmas and risks – for example:

◆ Those **not** sharing the targeted identity – who are not Black or gay or female – may underestimate the working connections and contributions they **can** make.

◆ As the agency specialises its responses through named workers 'over there', the non-specialists attending to their own apparently separate business 'over here' may begin to act as if all that needs to be done **is** being done within the organisation about this form of discrimination. Unequal and oppressive practices which persist **throughout** its provision, and not least within their own specialisms, may then not get recognised.

◆ All this may result in organisational fragmentation and a further marginalisation within the agency of the very issues which the named posts were designated to address in the first place.

42nd Street has lived through such processes in some very real ways. Initially, for example, its specialist Suicide and Self-harm Project took on much of the agency's work on suicide and self-harm. The same seemed to be happening in its responses to gay, lesbian and bisexual young people. Yet each now works with young people whose access to the agency was via the other, have highlighted the needs of both groups and have striven to create a climate of respect between them. Out of these processes have come clear expectations that all in the agency have a responsibility for taking on the relevant issues, with the necessary awareness and commitments coming to permeate throughout the organisation.

In a second contradictory twist, 42nd Street's history can be taken to suggest that an active celebration of diversity can also, over time, threaten to overlay, and even to some extent neutralise, the very features which it was intended to embed within the agency's programmes and culture. As in any organisation, within 42nd Street these exert on those caught within its net – young people and volunteers no less than workers and RMC members – their own in-built pressures to greater conformity and uniformity and in favour of a steady equilibrium. Once settled within this culture, even the organisation's more challenging initiatives, including those concerned with fulfilling a commitment to equal opportunities which positively embraces difference, can become established as acceptable and normal. The contention and the risk which were the essence of their original rationale may then be reduced or even deactivated or suppressed so that, as one Black worker noted, *'what's distinctive about what I do gets incorporated into 42nd Street's dominant culture'*.

Yet, to deliver their defining distinctiveness, such contributions need, sometimes abrasively, to rub up against established organisational ways of thinking and practising. Perversely, too benign or unproblematic an acceptance of what makes diversity diverse and distinctiveness distinct can mean that each loses its edginess – and therefore its vital edge. The agency's internal dynamics may then become less sensitive or responsive to the nonconformity which gives it its definition.

These dilemmas are now part of 42nd Street's ongoing (self) critical debate on implementing its equal opportunities commitments, particularly to embracing difference. One Black volunteer, for example, commented on how *'my Blackness can be relegated to insignificance, till it ceases to be an issue'*. A Black worker reflected: *'I often feel assimilated into the agency's culture, to a certain kind of approach, to the point where my Blackness is ignored. Workers can lose what they brought with them so this isn't as valued as it was.'*

Such reactions, it needs to be reiterated, are, of course, only one side of a complex equation, including for most of those actually raising the questions. In the discussion which produced them, for example, another participant confirmed what was said earlier about the impact of specialisms on generalist provision; *'the work with gay, lesbian and bisexual young people started like that (by employing named workers) – and look how comfortable they are now in 42nd Street'*. This view was endorsed, too, by at least one referring agency anxious to emphasise the levels of security and non-judgmental acceptance achieved by gay, lesbian and bisexual young people within 42nd Street and the gains this brought to them for tackling their related mental health problems.

Some oppressions more equal than others?

Another of the dilemmas even of progress towards an effective equal opportunities practice was highlighted by the referring agency which reported that *'one young man we referred to 42nd Street didn't go back because the worker who interviewed him was gay'*. While homophobic incidents were not unknown, one worker commented specifically on the agency's *'in-your-face attitude to sexuality'*, prompting another to advocate *'prejudicial starting points in favour of straight young men'*. Such apparent blocks to young straight men's involvement add additional weight to the arguments which had already led to the establishment of a specialist men's project aimed at responding to the growing evidence of young men's emotional and psychological vulnerability.

Nor was sexual identity the only focus of tensions between 'the oppressions', certainly amongst users. While the *StreetCred?* consultations were in progress, male sensitivities were bruised by a blunt 'aren't men a pain?' message appearing on the noticeboard of a recently formed women's-only group. Some of the young men affected in fact displayed higher levels of awareness than might normally have been expected of why the young women might be saying such things, accepting their right – and need – to assert themselves, not least against their treatment by men. Nonetheless, for one (male) worker, in a context where male users' self-esteem was often already pretty low, there were genuine worries that *'once again the young men coming to 42nd Street have been defined as bad objects'*. Staff concerns were expressed, too, that some (albeit unintended) encouragement was being given to an unhelpful competitiveness between male and female users.

Efforts to negotiate more appropriate interventions with other marginalised or excluded groups also regularly bumped into each other. How, for example, to achieve a greater responsiveness to suicide and self-harm without conveying the unintended message that other concerns had lower status, including even perhaps young people's experiences of abuse. Or, as one RMC asked: *'How to get to work on homophobia and masculinity with Black young men which goes beyond racist perceptions and definitions of them and their attitudes.'*

What cumulatively the 42nd Street experience would therefore seem to demonstrate is that the very arrival, and then the search for security, of one excluded group can churn up eddies of disturbance. These can then buffet the equilibrium of others who – often with long histories of marginalisation elsewhere – have established their foothold at 42nd Street. Meanwhile, interweaving with such tensions are important developmental and liberating effects – as when a group of white users, told that many Black young people feel uncertain about coming to 42nd Street, responded with: 'Take us to meet them. We'll convince 'em.'

The equal opportunities balance sheet

When equal opportunities is the issue, as smoothly as in any area of an agency's policy and practice, slogans can rule and confrontation with the struggles to make these real may be evaded or denied. Yet for caring, person-centred organisations like 42nd Street rooted in the best liberal traditions of the voluntary sector of the British welfare state, some cherished values may need some critical reappraisal. As was suggested earlier, uncompromising confrontation with destructively oppressive attitudes and behaviour may, for example, make it impossible to sustain an unreconstructed commitment to open-mindedness and tolerance of others' (bigoted) views. It can also cut against the grain of valued 'organic' **processes** of human interaction. Have people's (discriminatory) starting points in their search for personal change always to be respected? Must this change always occur at their own (discriminatory) pace, working from their (at time oppressive) strengths, emphasising reward and avoiding blame and punishment?

How in fact do you balance, on the one hand, recognition of an individual or group's need, in their own way and in their own time, to deal with their prejudices and exploitative responses to others; with, on the other, offering protection from the hurt (or worse) which in the process they may be causing their targets?

Ultimately, in fact, the tripping phrases in support of tackling discrimination and oppression mask an uncomfortable 'zero sum' phenomenon. To deliver on them requires some redistribution of finite amounts of **power**, from those who have it and are usually reluctant to give up its advantages to those whose lack of it leaves them consistently – institutionally – marginalised.

42nd Street has often had to learn through experience where and how the slogans, with intent or otherwise, can gloss over these complexities. What this experience has particularly clarified is that there is no substitute for 'going for it' – for making specific and concrete commitments (not least resource commitments). Moreover, these need to be to tackling not just gaps in provision but the gaps in individual and collective awareness into which often unnoticed discriminatory cultural norms and practices are liable to insinuate themselves and exercise great influence.

Such an approach will inevitably produce some (often no win) situations which it is not easy – probably not possible – for any organisation to avoid altogether. These, however, cannot be used as excuses or even reasons for backing off when the complexities of the slogans start to unravel. What 42nd Street's history reveals is that, far from being seen as unfortunate accidents, they have to be treated as intrinsic elements of the equal opportunities commitment itself – and that policy development, practice and training must therefore be planned accordingly.

Chapter 6: Internal culture and external relations

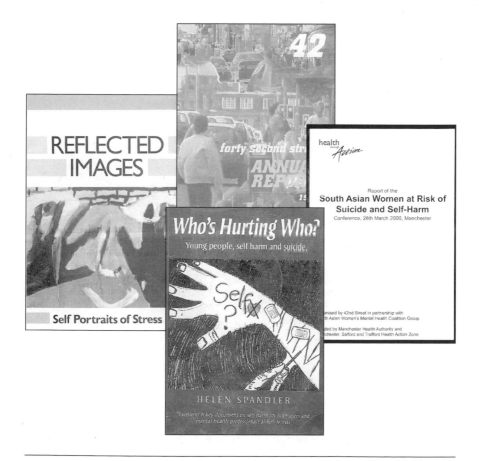

Chapter 6: Internal culture and external relations

42ⁿᵈ Street in its wider context

42ⁿᵈ Street's history has run parallel to huge changes in the funding environment of all voluntary organisations. From the (in retrospect) generosity and stability of historic grant-aid arrangements and five-year Urban Aid allocations, it now has to pick its way through the mysteries of service agreements and contracts, demands for voluntary-statutory partnerships, outcome funding initiatives and annually renewable grants. Like any other voluntary body, it also finds itself negotiating a roller-coaster of bids to the National Lottery, Comic Relief, the Diana Fund and private trusts, to say nothing of bodies such as the National Youth Agency and the Mental Health Foundation. As it has expanded into Salford and Trafford, equally complex funding arrangements have had to be negotiated with local councils and health authorities.

As its annual turnover and expansion show (see below), in making these shifts 42ⁿᵈ Street has prospered in comparison to many other agencies. It has done so, moreover, even though in 1990, in somewhat fraught circumstances, it separated from its original sponsor, the Youth Development Trust. Since then, the Resource Management Committee's belief in, and commitment to, the agency have been crucial in providing the vital link for holding together the internal and external worlds and thereby ensuring its public credibility. At the same time, the committee has clearly worked hard to make its own operational style and methods congruent with 42ⁿᵈ Street's overall commitment to worker and user participation. As work pressures among the potential target groups make the recruitment of volunteer members to voluntary organisation management committees increasingly difficult, the maintenance of this group as an effective working entity is still very far from straightforward.

Indeed, more widely, the relatively secure position reached by 42nd Street by the end of the 1990s was not achieved without strain. It is, after all, an agency which attracts highly committed individuals, sometimes on salaries below those of the statutory sector, who come to 42nd Street on the at least implicit condition that it deliver on its value commitments. With most giving high priority to being as articulate as possible about their ideological starting points, they can therefore be relentless in resisting any perceived deviations from these. In negotiating the twisting funding tracks of the past decade and more, 42nd Street has proved to be both extremely agile and philosophically focused – a balancing act which, as the fate of other voluntary organisations has shown, is very far from straightforward. Indeed, as we shall see in the next chapter, on such issues a value-driven agency like 42nd Street is as likely to implode as to achieve compromise with integrity.

In fact, though often extremely uncomfortable, such value-driven conflicts would seem to have helped to keep 42nd Street on its toes by prompting constant self-scrutiny. One of the key focuses of this has been ensuring that the agency's internal environment has remained responsive to fast-changing external expectations. Here above all 42nd Street seems to have identified sources of renewable intellectual and practice energy which have not just sustained it through very trying times. They have also enabled it to go on evolving in ways which are right for its crucial constituency – young people experiencing often severe emotional and psychological stress – in the process influencing strategic thinking both locally and nationally. It has, for example, played a critical role in placing the needs of 14 to 25-year-olds on local health authority agendas, while its developing model for work with young people who have attempted suicide and who self-harm is increasingly recognised as meriting wider replication.

Not collectivity but participation

Walking the internal-external tightrope has perhaps been at its most testing as increasingly 42nd Street has been required to balance its commitment to significant degrees of staff, volunteer and user participation in decision-making with meeting shifting contractual demands for 'hard' objectives, milestones and outcome and output measures. In this negotiation, particularly to be in good shape to survive as an independent organisation, it has abandoned its earlier non-hierarchical team arrangements in which all in a six-person team were paid the same and carried equal responsibility for running the organisation. In its place it has, over time, instituted an (albeit very flat) hierarchical (and explicit) **management** structure which now provides for two coordinators, two practice managers and an office and resources manager.

Nonetheless, participation has remained a core 42nd Street principle. As we saw in Chapter 4, this has particularly high profile in its direct work with young people: indeed, despite charity commissioners' scepticism, it was formally embodied in the 42nd Street constitution at the time of its separation from the Youth Development Trust. It is integral, too, to the roles of workers and even of volunteers, all of which are seen as carrying significant responsibility for planning and developing as well as actually delivering 42nd Street's services to young people.

As with young people's participation, here too the notion tends often to have a strong constitutional connotation, focusing on where and how key internal actors (paid and unpaid) fit into the governance of the organisation through representation on the RMC and other decision-making arenas. It is also still played out very clearly in team meetings – now of course much larger and more numerous and varied than 20 years ago. In these, consideration of operational management matters allows a wide range of workers to contribute to decisions which in other organisations would, after being taken by those in more senior managerial roles, often simply be communicated down the line. These processes also often display a taken-for-granted colleagueship – for example, in the understanding and support offered both staff and young people going on the Amsterdam and Slovenia trips (see Chapter 4) – which contains it own messages about organisational cohesion and collectivity.

Within 42nd Street, centralised hierarchical structures, mechanisms and processes are thus still rejected – in action as often as in words – in favour of ones which spread involvement and ownership as widely as is feasible. Where these do not extend to actually taking the necessary decisions, they, as a minimum, bring advice on what should be done. In addition to team meetings, key forums achieving this have included working groups, away days for reflecting on broader policy issues and in 2000 a process for producing a five-year plan which involved young people, volunteers, workers and RMC members.

It is at least implicit here too that, for such participation to be credible and effective, it must percolate beyond formal decision-making into daily practice and management. Again this reveals itself most clearly in a variety of team and sub-team meetings used for sharing practice experience, sometimes in considerable detail. For some, the very process of the *StreetCred?* consultations sparked comments on how rarely workers (and presumably others) met just to analyse practice and draw out its wider philosophical and policy lessons. Though, it is true, the established mechanisms within 42nd Street normally allowed limited scope for this, to an outsider such structured-in debates still appeared more extensive and more probing than in most similar organisations. These proceeded, what is more, on a set of given norms in favour of open and honest self and team appraisal, of feelings as well as of facts, which was also far from routine. One former worker reflected for example that: *'There's a culture here of taking the work seriously. There's time to reflect – to think about the impact on me … I learned a lot, developed, gained confidence.'* A funder commented: *'This is a critical moment for voluntary organisations. 42nd Street needs its openness, its genuineness.'*

In part this commitment to operational participation may be driven by practical realities: after all, disempowered staff are unlikely to have much energy or incentive to empower users and may well end up **de**motivated about much else, too. However, much more principled considerations on staff participation are at work here. A commitment to a practice which respects individuals, their rights and their abilities is seen as needing to be underpinned by what might be called worker-centred relations with and between staff of all kinds. Thus 42nd Street aspires to an organisational culture which allows **and supports** workers and volunteers to act with considerable (perhaps risk-taking) discretion and autonomy in their agreed areas of activity. It also assumes they will contribute to the wider processes of maintaining and developing the agency.

At first sight such a philosophy and the practical arrangements flowing from it can look like one of those simplistic rejections of hierarchical structures which characterised many of the 'alternative' voluntary and community organisations which, like 42nd Street, emerged out of the 1970s and early 1980s. Significantly, one analysis of these, published in 1985 [13], dubbed them a 'radical failure' and was uncompromising in its dismissal of such idealist organisational strategies. It concluded that *'undefined responsibility is too lightly undertaken without considering the nature of the job or whether ... (this) is the right person to do it'*, thereby in effect defining the skill of management as *'merely to stop people bumping into each other'*. The resultant power vacuums then had to be filled by informal and often unacknowledged processes leading to *'a kind of de facto policy-making'*. As all this rested, too, on an ignorance of how the external system works, relations with key and powerful outside bodies often became distorted and even unsustainable.

As its movement to its current management structures shows, 42nd Street has very self-consciously learnt and applied the lessons of such failures, in the process explicitly distancing itself from simplistic notions of collectivity. All the key groups involved in its work, including on occasions users, place tough conditions and limits on their commitments to participation. These emphasise the need for appropriate boundaries for people and activities, clear and agreed roles for all the main interest groups and the individuals within them, and specified lines of accountability.

Thus, to meet positive developmental objectives rather than merely for reasons of containment, users' behaviour is guided very specifically through widely publicised ground rules. Parallel staff parameters are embodied – and in part for not altogether dissimilar developmental reasons – in regular supervision with line managers and in formal appraisals. As we saw earlier, though the tensions

[13] Charles Landry et al, *What a Way to Run a Railroad*, Comedia, 1985.

can often be severe and sometimes abrasive, 42nd Street's negotiation of an at times unsympathetic external environment is conducted on the basis that, far from just being repudiated, this has its own rationales which had better be understood and respected. Nor is this done only to win funding or agree service contracts. In 1996 the external evaluation of 42nd Street's Education Project concluded that – in part *'by knowing and insisting on their own clear value-driven approach'* – the project's workers had *'had to develop the ability to go into "alien" institutions and be credible with both staff and young people'*. [14]

Gaps and dilemmas in a participative culture

However, in striving to be neither oppressively authoritarian nor naively or unrealistically democratic, 42nd Street again finds itself having to confront and negotiate a number of dilemmas and tensions. The implications of these for relations with young people have been considered throughout this book. This chapter concentrates primarily on their significance for 42nd Street as a collective and institutional entity which is greater than the sum of its parts. It also examines its implications for those – volunteers, paid staff and RMC members – with a primary responsibility for planning, managing and delivering its services.

Is bigger beautiful?

One question which repeatedly surfaces in discussions about 42nd Street's development and future is: can its distinctive value-driven style, approach and culture survive as it gets bigger and its structures become more elaborate?

In 1986, the 42nd Street staff comprised six full-time and three part-time workers. At that time some 10 volunteers were involved in its work and it was catering for approximately two hundred young people. Throughout this initial period of development it operated effectively as a small collective.

---

[14] *New Wine in Old Bottles*, Youth Work Press, 1996.

In 1987 42nd Street introduced an (extremely flat) management structure in which two joint coordinators supervised all staff in their work with young people. At the time this study was completed 42nd Street employed twenty full-time and ten part-time staff. Eighteen volunteers were involved and the number of users had increased to over seven hundred a year. While the *StreetCred?* consultations were in progress an extra tier of management was added with the appointment of two practice managers with responsibility for supervising some fieldwork staff and overseeing other agency-wide tasks such as volunteer coordination and suicide and self-harm work. The business of the RMC had expanded and become much more complex, not least in order to exercise control over a total annual budget of £730,000.

In safeguarding the essential 42nd Street value base, the dilemmas here seemed to many within the organisation to be stark. Getting bigger simply for the sake of getting bigger cannot be justified – though the temptations here can be considerable at a time when voluntary sector organisations, especially in the mental health field, are increasingly being put under pressure to provide total community-based services. (Indeed, 42nd Street has had on occasions to resist precisely such blandishments, in at least one instance offering instead consultancy support to statutory sector colleagues so they could provide the service themselves.)

On the other hand, expansion has clearly in recent years proved justified, even inescapable, in order to respond to young people's changing needs and to the growing stress and deepening despair which so many of them are experiencing. It has been justified, too, in order to win financial backing for the distinctive responses, alternative to those normally available through statutory services, which mark out 42nd Street's way of working.

But what if the built-in consequences of such expansion undermine what has made 42nd Street 'alternative'? What if such growth is incompatible with its person-centred and participative culture? What if it requires more tiers of management and the inevitable distancing from decision-making for many staff that this would bring? Though the addition of two further managerial posts has been accepted within the agency as the best workable compromise available, typically few within 42nd Street seem to assume that this particular debate has been resolved.

Who can participate?

Even within its present parameters, however, 42nd Street's participative structures and processes seemed to be hitting some realistic buffers. These perhaps show up most clearly in the roles and status which volunteers and part-time workers are able to achieve within the organisation.

Volunteers undertake a range of responsibilities, including, for example, working in the drop-in, facilitating members' meetings and, most notably, acting as befrienders including helping users to come to the agency, get to college or attend a sports centre. All the eight volunteers consulted for the *StreetCred?* project gave overwhelmingly positive assessments of their experience at 42nd Street. They were clear that *'volunteers are really respected'*; that *'the role of volunteers here is treated very seriously'*; even that *'being a volunteer here can be transforming'*. One said: *'I came to get experience and for my CV – but I just stayed.'*

They particularly approved of 42nd Street's volunteer recruitment procedures, training, induction and support programmes. These they described as *'impressive, very effective, very involving, very real, very challenging personally, very refreshing in comparison with the social work course I'm doing'*. Here again the agency's clarity about its values and purposes and the consistency with which these were to be applied caught their attention. One commented: *'It has a clear value base which has remained with me. It's refreshing to come back here from the individualistic approaches of (another agency).'* Another concluded that *'though most of the values are implicit … they're the key to 42nd Street'* while a third added *'(though) the values are very deliberately explored during recruitment … they're not imposed – they're not a rigid set of rules'*.

As we saw in earlier chapters, volunteers felt clear, too, about their roles in the agency's overall provision of services, unapologetically seeing themselves as *'second in line'* and accepting that *'the power relations are with the workers'*. They were also able to recognise the advantages in such divisions of labour, suggesting, for example, that *'young people are more open with us ... we're a bridge between worker and young person'*.

However, this sense of a genuine involvement in practice and of owning their role as volunteer **workers** has to be set alongside the constraints on wider volunteer participation within 42nd Street. These not only restricted their contributions to team and other collective activities. They could also leave them relatively isolated and contributing in individualistic ways, *'as befrienders largely operating behind the scenes'* (worker); *'in and out of the agency'* (worker); *'with no sense of collective involvement'* (volunteer); *'individually very committed and with a lot of good ideas but they can't be active'* (worker).

Appointing a full-time staff member with responsibility for volunteer coordination has been 42nd Street's way of trying to break down these limitations. Yet, as one worker with managerial responsibilities pointed out, like other organisations using volunteers 42nd Street is facing *'a structural problem'* defined by the narrowly specified amounts and periods of time volunteers can offer for undertaking some equally narrowly delineated forms of work.

The situation of part-time paid workers is not quite as stark. As one worker recognised: *'Part-timers give real value for money. Per unit cost they are very productive. For face-to-face contact they're doing very much the same job as full-timers. Expectations of part timers are as high as for full-timers.'*

And the external evaluation of the agency's Education Project concluded: *'The staffing structure of one full-time ... and four part-time staff has benefited the project through the variety of skills and experiences available in terms of gender, race and sexuality ... Sessional (part-time) workers have been full members of the team ... and have made vitally important contributions.'* [15]

Nonetheless, the structural position of part-timers also produces tensions,

---

[15] *New Wine in Old Bottles*, Youth Work Press, 1996, p.15.

rooted, in their case, in real contractual and indeed financial constraints with one (full-time) worker, for example, noting: *'Team work for part-timers is very difficult ... they may have only limited contact.'*

Who gains from participation – and who loses?

As we saw earlier in this chapter, a striking feature of the 42nd Street culture is the implicit and explicit support it gives to open debate about the work, both in general and with a focus on individuals' own work. This was occurring in an unusually wide range of public arenas – team and sub-team meetings, training sessions, away-days, committee and subcommittee meetings, though the emphasis on personal supervision, both managerial and non-managerial, suggested to some workers something of a drift towards a 'privatisation' of practice.

The personal and professional exposure which almost unavoidably comes with such participative processes and structures can, anyway, set up its own strains. For one thing, deviance, however mild and inconsequential for the work, can become more public. As one former worker recalled: *'42nd Street's is a culture which takes itself seriously – lots of self-reflection, what's the impact on this or that for me? I had a deviant office – noisy, where we had a laugh, untidy. It didn't quite fit the 42nd Street image.'*

Secondly, the openness produced by 42nd Street's participative style can, albeit unintentionally, exacerbate the self-doubt about professional identities and skills discussed in Chapter 3, especially in a multi-disciplinary setting. After all this is organisational ground which offers staff fewer than normal sheltering places. One worker, for example had discovered that: *'42nd Street is very open in its recruitment process – it values experience as well as qualifications. Everything's then up for grabs – you have an anxiety: "Am I living up to 42nd Street's standards?"'*

Looking back, a former worker wondered: *'Do the pressures and tensions of working at 42nd Street help or hinder workers, especially younger workers? You ask: "What have I to offer young people? How do I do that?"'*

Indeed another former worker, reflecting on what (if anything) was unique about 42nd Street and on the reality behind *'its mystique for outsiders'*, suggested that: *'New workers can feel very insecure about meeting 42nd Street's standards and expectations. I feel I never really cracked the mystery.'* This worker was even left wondering whether, with its carefully cultivated internal culture of mutual support and staff ownership of decisions, 42nd Street might not have insulated itself from some valid reality tests. These included those messy organisational processes and interfaces which help give agencies a 'fix' on the outside world and keep its collective feet on the ground. Albeit in a way which seemed to under-estimate 42nd Street's own pressures from insistent unplanned demand, the difference for this ex-worker seemed to be encapsulated in a contrast with an agency which had *'all those young people in very immediate crisis constantly banging on the door'*.

But – does distinctiveness count? Do values pay?

Such views, it needs perhaps to be reiterated, were more than matched by very positive assessments of the way 42nd Street conducted its business and relationships internally and externally. Moreover, these came not just, repeatedly, from current paid staff but also from the range of other interests within and without 42nd Street.

For example, one user commented: *'Other organisations put young people down ... I feel a young person but am treated like an adult ...but can be a young person if I like. I can't do that anywhere else.'*

From a former worker came the comment: *'It's certain to go on attracting funds because it's confident about its identity and gets a proper user view. Its marketing is good because it's clear about what it's got to sell, what it does, and it can explain it. Its commitment to participation is a real strength – not just tokenistic.'*

And from an admin worker: *'We can usually decide for funders what the important evaluation questions are. This comes from workers' confidence in what they're doing.'*

Particularly significantly given what was said at the start of this chapter about 42nd Street's undisguised and unapologetic **value-driven** pitch for its resources seemed to be the views of funders:

> '42nd Street is an "alternative" organisation – flexible and unique in its way of attracting young people ... It deals with a group of young people not dealt with by a social services department. It offers some unique roles – without having that social services overlay.'

> '42nd Street knows what it is doing and can resist tempting funding offers which could undermine its role. It has to jar on occasions with the local authority – it's an alternative voice. There'd be something wrong if it didn't. It's clearly within the partnership ... but it represents its distinctiveness very clearly and strongly. It's strong in knowing its core business ...'

> 'It's an organisation ... which has a "can-do" culture. Not a "don't know" culture like some other voluntary organisations.'

Standing up to be counted

The health, educational and welfare worlds continue to need a strong voluntary sector of this kind. At a time when the state is seeking to entice voluntary organisations into a closer and closer embrace, they particularly need agencies like 42nd Street – striving to be clear about their values, unafraid of asserting these and yet unafraid, too, of acknowledging the paradoxes posed and the inconsistencies to be mediated.

Precisely because – as the 42nd Street experience also shows – these dilemmas infiltrate policy-making and management as sharply as they do practice, their negotiation requires internal structures and processes which can win the widest possible ownership within the organisation, including among users. This is needed, too, to underpin an engagement with the external political and funding environment which can be assured, robust and, where necessary, uncompromising, especially on behalf of users and their access to services. Where these users are young people – and, what is more, young people experiencing severe stress and even breakdown – such strength is particularly needed. Above all it is required to ensure that the provision which results goes beyond mechanistic 'treatments' to espousing, as 42nd Street has sought to do, empowering forms of therapy, support and individual and collective expression.

Chapter 7: Managing choices in a value-driven organisation

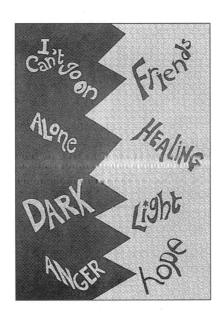

Chapter 7: Managing choices in a value-driven organisation

Ambiguous values

A key aim of this book has been to illustrate and illuminate the choices and dilemmas facing an agency like 42nd Street which is powerfully and self-consciously driven by the values it espouses. Here, after all, is a voluntary organisation which exists to address an issue – mental health – whose value content is, to say the least, ambiguous. Indeed, with key players often masking or denying this content, 'patients' encountering related organisations – sometimes left with few, if any, choices – are most often still treated for 'symptoms' based on 'diagnoses' which continue to be run through with high degrees of subjectivity.

Interweaving with this core set of value issues are others which, for all health, education and welfare agencies, contain their own considerable ambiguity. For example:

◆ Who do these agencies choose to include in their category of young people; why them; and how far even before that of 'mentally ill' has been added, does this label in itself stigmatise and exclude?

◆ How far do such agencies adopt a minimalist definition of equal opportunities and anti-discrimination with difference grudgingly accommodated as, in effect, a deviance from dominant norms? Or do they positively assert the value of such diversity both to the individual and to society, seeking in the process to nurture and strengthen it?

◆ Do they even recognise young people's right to and need for participation? Insofar as they do, how far do they see such empowerment as an (again grudging) concession – to be made in this case to ensure the young's more effective management and socialisation? Or do they embrace and encourage empowerment as both a practical recognition of young people's capacity and right to self-determination and, again, as a contribution to the social good?

In the case of 42nd Street a further set of value questions arise because of its choice to adopt forms of service delivery, policy-making and management which, from staff as well as users, seek maximum participation and consensus. This is most clearly seen in its internal consultative and decision-making arrangements which emphasise as wide a spread of involvement and contribution as is compatible with providing a focused and accountable service to young people. But it is at least implicit, too, in its development of a multi-disciplinary model of practice which by its very nature requires a range of transparent personal and professional exchanges among all those working in the agency.

A framework for understanding 'values issues'

Such dilemmas are not of course special to 42nd Street. In a trenchant analysis of the potential impact of such 'values issues' in voluntary agencies[16], Rob Paton in effect cautions that they have two common, even if not essential, characteristics. They usually generate strong feelings; and they are *'inherently prone to escalate, which may happen rapidly, leading to polarisation and even irreconcilable differences, expulsions or splits'.*

None of the evidence from the *StreetCred?* consultations in any way suggested that 42nd Street is facing these kinds of disruption or disintegration. On the contrary, despite sometimes being personally uncomfortable and occasionally inhibiting for the organisation, its internal debates more often lend support to Paton's thesis that such dialogue and indeed soul-searching is for 42nd Street instrumental *'in maintaining the aspirations of the organisation'.*

---

[16] Rob Paton, 'How are Values Handled in Voluntary Agencies?', in D. Billis and M. Morris (eds.) *Voluntary Agencies*, 1996.

Nonetheless, Paton's framework for examining value-driven voluntary organisations does repeatedly seem to speak very directly to 42nd Street's 20-year experience. Paton suggests that value conflicts occur because, particularly in small or medium-sized organisations which operate through more informal internal processes, values and commitments *'are more likely to be ambiguous and hence open to conflicting interpretations'*. He points out, too, that: *'To the extent that many voluntary organisations are participatively and consensually managed, they provide more opportunities for value issues to emerge and flare up.'*

Paton also draws the specific conclusion that: *'... rows and disputes over values issues in the course of day-to-day activities arise more often in radical and campaigning voluntary organisations than in traditional service-delivery voluntary organisations or public sector organisations.'*

These disputes are most commonly expressed as disagreements over:

◆ what the commitments actually mean;

◆ how to achieve consistency between them and the action they require; and

◆ what the relative priority should be among different commitments.

Most importantly, in developing this analysis, Paton makes clear that *'some inconsistency between values and action is inevitable – indeed it may even be desirable in maintaining the aspirations of the organisation'*. He also points out that *'argument may not be reducible to "managerial judgment" ... a utilitarian calculus of costs and benefits'* since, though often confronted as if it were right against wrong, what is often actually at stake is **right against right**. Certainly, one of the clearest and potentially most far-reaching of the lessons of this study of 42nd Street's value base and dilemmas is echoed in Paton's conclusion that: *'The inevitability of values issues arising means that they cannot be seen as embarrassing aberrations or a sign of management failure ... Values issues may be more or less successfully handled, but they cannot be avoided – except, perhaps, by having less thoughtful and committed staff and volunteers.'*

Some outstanding values issues and questions for 42nd Street

Given the thought and commitment invested in its work by its staff and volunteers, avoidance of its unresolved values issues has hardly been an option for 42nd Street. A number of such issues have been picked out by this study, including some (though not all) which can only be described as ongoing – even sometimes long-running – sagas.

◆ In its *conceptualisations of youth and adolescence*, notions of **transitions** emphasising young people's preparation to become the adults we wish them to be seem at times to be operating most explicitly and therefore perhaps more influentially within 42nd Street. This would suggest that the importance to young people of **their here and now** expectations and experiences might merit clearer and more frequent articulation.

◆ In *conceptualising 'mental health'*, 42nd Street would seem still to have some work to do to clarify what it means by a **social model**, what the political content and implications of this might be and how these might percolate more actively into its policy and practice.

◆ If some retrospective as well as occasionally current evaluations are any guide, sustaining *a multi-disciplinary approach* is likely to need continuing **affirmation of the core professional identities** which workers bring with them to 42nd Street. It may also need to go on clarifying some **methodological boundaries** and particularly the 'fit' of 42nd Street's conception of informal support for individual young people with the core methods of counselling, group work and developmental youth work.

◆ In sustaining its commitment to *young people's participation*, continuing vigilance is going to be needed, too, to ensure that this remains **open to the generality of members** rather than becoming settled on a particular (perhaps elite) group of users. Striking the **balance between user participation and organisational (particularly RMC) efficiency** also seems likely to remain a concern which will run and run.

◆ In the context of its value position on *equal opportunities*, for some within 42nd Street, **consciousness of class** and how it shapes (and constrains) young people's lives remains underdeveloped – certainly when compared to the open and consistent focus put on other social divisions. Many would add too that, again given these comparisons, the agency's heightened **consciousness of disability** has developed rather late.

◆ For maintaining its commitment to *consultative and participatory internal processes*, 42nd Street's dilemma over **whether bigger can continue to be beautiful** is unlikely to evaporate. Within this, questions about the fuller **involvement of volunteers and part-time workers** will almost certainly persist as will, here too, ones about the protection of core professional identities within its often exposing staff structures.

Values issues, service delivery and management: some lessons from 42nd Street's experience

For addressing such outstanding values issues, policy-making, planning and service delivery within 42nd Street seem to start from the premise that, because neither the goals nor the processes for reaching these are one-dimensional, potential value compromises have to be confronted openly. Notwithstanding the gaps and work-in-progress outlined above, this has helped to prevent value differences from going subterranean and oo becoming subversive.

Service delivery

And so, for example, in relation to issues impinging most directly on how the agency's service is delivered to young people:

◆ 42nd Street has not just stood on the sidelines philosophically sniping at the medical model of mental health or, even more risky, getting drawn into opportunistic hit and run skirmishes with its advocates. Nor, because they are there, has it just grudgingly reconciled itself to dealing with conventional psychiatry and its treatments. Rather, while insisting on the universality and primacy of mental **health** even among its large proportion of users with serious emotional and psychological problems, it has made the conscious and carefully targeted choice to infiltrate the heart of the beast. Thus, it has offered consultancy services to statutory agencies on community-based provision and, via outreach approaches, drawing on its own research findings, it has piloted alternative models of work within local hospitals for young people who have attempted suicide or who self-harm.

◆ In maintaining a young people-centred focus, 42nd Street has explicitly distanced itself from assumptions that this is the same as young people-led. Indeed, it openly advances the view that an ultimate authority has to be **held** by workers, albeit 'helpfully'. Alongside this, it has embraced the notion of boundaried practice, as a safeguard against idealist commitments to young people whose lives are often highly disorganised and whose self-esteem and confidence can be at rock bottom.

◆ In pursuing participation, ground rules are explicitly laid down and proactively worked with so that promises of power are not made to young people – for example, over involvement in appointing staff or spending money – which cannot be delivered. This includes avoiding setting goals which young people cannot realistically achieve given their individual starting points and stage of development or within their time commitment to 42nd Street.

◆ In pursuing equal opportunities, specialist (named) posts and projects have been created crucially but not only to open up access to specific identity groups for whom 42nd Street would not be an automatic or immediately comfortable port of call. These have been developed, too, as a lever on **all** staff, volunteers and (yet again) users to step up the agency's efforts to, in non-competitive ways, ensure such group's inclusion and affirmation.

Managing values issues

Drawing on Paton's analysis of value-driven voluntary organisations, 42nd Street's experience of **managing** values issues reflects other lessons which would seem to have a potentially wider resonance.

◆ Though it does not do to romanticise value issues, within 42nd Street these are approached positively, to encourage what Paton calls *'double-loop learning' – 'opportunities for inventing creative solutions that will allow an agency better to pursue its mission'.*

◆ As the contribution of 'an instrumentally rational approach' will be limited, other responses to these issues are often made on the basis that *'we are in the realm of politics and value-expressive behaviour, rather than administration'.* Small 'p' **political** skills are therefore seen as an important part of effective voluntary sector leadership in this area.

◆ Because *'many values issues involve irresolvable conflicts between right and right'* which have a tendency to escalate and polarise, *'how the issue is handled will often be more important than the particular decision which emerges'.* The medium of resolution or accommodation then becomes an integral part of the final message.

In other words, as Paton points out: *'... protecting, developing and negotiating the meaning of values, in order to preserve a more or less viable set of commitments, needs to be recognised as a crucial part of management in many voluntary agencies'*

– and, many would add, in statutory agencies, too.

Though again they have not been without their ambiguities and even contradictions, in striving to meet such expectations, 42nd Street's efforts to establish and then adapt consultative and participative structures for decision-making would seem to have been crucial. Involvement in such decision-making has been spread unusually wide in order to secure no less unusual degrees of internal ownership of what the agency is doing. At the same time, again deliberately, significant checks on and balances against presumptions of collectivity have been built into the way the organisation steers itself strategically and manages itself day-to-day. These have been seen as essential in part to ensure that 42nd Street's interface with an increasingly complex and demanding outside world – funders, partners in service delivery, referral agencies – is clearly delineated, credible and efficient. They have been required, too, to provide unambiguous and effective internal lines of accountability and support for both workers and volunteers which, while underpinning this external credibility, are above all capable of carrying the weight of catering to a vulnerable and needy clientele.

Restless minds and renewable energies

Over its 20-year history, 42nd Street has managed to negotiate a very delicate balancing act. On the one hand it has largely remained **un**polarised, has avoided irreconcilable splits and so has maintained its stability. On the other, populated by enough restless minds to remain unwilling to settle for where it has reached, it has stayed responsive to change in young people's lives and in the wider (especially funding) environment in which it must move. As one volunteer put it: *'It **has never grown old – never become fuddy duddy.'**

To a significant degree, it has generated and then drawn repeatedly on these renewable sources of organisational energy. Often – though not, of course, always – it has done this by working deliberately **with** rather than against the grain of the tensions inherent in its value choices (and compromises), choosing to embrace and even open up these tensions as essential stimulants to developing effective and realistic practice.

The result is that only exceptionally does 42nd Street seem to find itself displacing its energies in diversionary and potentially debilitating struggles over secondary issues – what procedures must be adopted to do this, who has the right to do that, whether something else might be bad for the agency's image. Of course, 42nd Street does not lack an internal personal and inter-personal politics – which organisation does? Most consistently, however, the focus of its main debates seems to remain firmly on its core commitment – to young people and to their mental health.

One contributor to the 1999 Annual Report expressed this central preoccupation very clearly: *'we think very deeply about mental health issues and ... have a lot to contribute ... So we keep constantly in mind that we want to make a positive difference to mental health services in this country, and to encourage other young people to make their voices heard through our work and participation at 42nd Street.'*

It seems wholly appropriate that, for capturing the essence of 42nd Street's philosophy and value base, this statement should have come from a user.

Members' Afterword

A group of young people met to discuss what was being said in this book. They recognised that they had influenced the production of the book through various meetings with the author. However, they decided that they would like to contribute a final section which would bring their own voices to a wider audience. They chose to comment on the following three topics.

1) *What it's like being a young person in the year 2000, and the pressures and stresses that young people face*

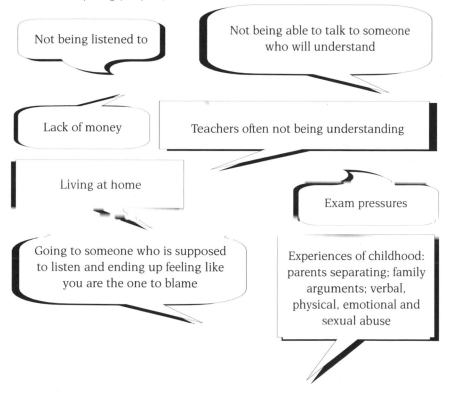

It's hard to get employment when you have to tell the employer about your mental health history

Being lied to by the Government about something like New Deal – that hasn't changed in the first place

The pressure of relationships – getting torn between friends and their relationships

Being young and not having control of your life – being treated like a child even though you're 15 or 16

Parents hiding secrets from you – being lied to by family

Being given too much responsibility at too young an age, for example, having to look after another family member when still only a child yourself

Family not understanding you

2) *Young people's experience of mental health in 2000*

Taking three weeks to get some medication off a doctor

Being treated like a joke by some members of the medical profession

Getting different medication from a doctor and feeling like a guinea pig

Depression and anxiety not being taken seriously

Going to Accident and Emergency and being treated like shit

Lack of knowledge and understanding about self harm by doctors and nurses

Workers saying that you'll grow out of it when you're feeling depressed

Or saying that you're too young to be depressed

It felt important that the psychiatrist was prepared to listen to me

Being treated like you're stupid because you're young

Being told that you need all those different people to help you

Not being told about the side effects of medication

People assuming that you are lazy because you've got mental health problems

3) *What is important about the services that 42nd Street offers?*

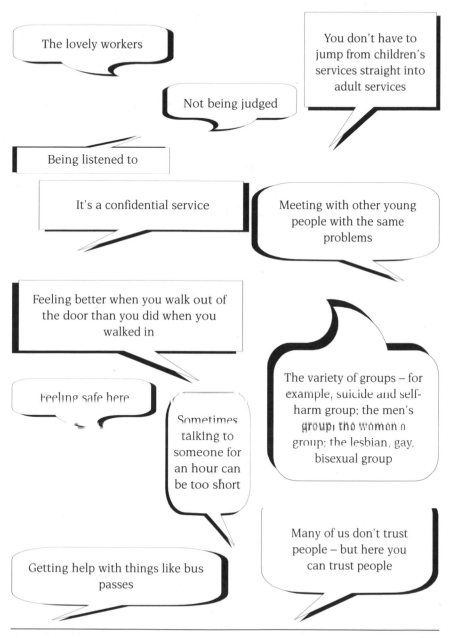

The lovely workers

You don't have to jump from children's services straight into adult services

Not being judged

Being listened to

It's a confidential service

Meeting with other young people with the same problems

Feeling better when you walk out of the door than you did when you walked in

Feeling safe here

Sometimes talking to someone for an hour can be too short

The variety of groups – for example, suicide and self-harm group; the men's group; the women's group; the lesbian, gay, bisexual group

Many of us don't trust people – but here you can trust people

Getting help with things like bus passes

The workers are usually young themselves – you can relate easily to them

Young people are involved in the running of the agency – you can get to say what you want and you get listened to, through members' meetings, management meetings and AGMs

Having access to computers is important – young people need access to the internet, for example, to get up-to-date information about suicide or self-harm; to talk to other agencies; to help young people in a group to write to other young people

Befriending help from volunteers is good for young people who can't get into 42nd Street for help

It was good that young people from the suicide and self-harm group organised and ran a suicide and self-harm awareness day for other agencies – which was very successful. It was sad that a young person had to miss this because she had to go into hospital that day

You've got somewhere to turn to when you need it

There could be better communication between young people and workers, and between workers and workers

More agencies should get young people involved in their services – it helps your mental health because it takes your mind off depression and other such problems